Clinical Techniques in Dentistry

Resin-Bonded Bridges

Clinical Techniques in Dentistry

Resin-Bonded Bridges

A Practitioner's Guide

WM Tay

PhD, BDS, FDSRCS

Reader in Conservative Dentistry
The London Hospital Medical College Dental School, UK

MARTIN DUNITZ

First published in 1992 by
Martin Dunitz Ltd, The Livery House, 7–9 Pratt Street, London NW1 0AE

A CIP catalogue record for this title is available from the British Library.

ISBN 0–948269–41–3

Composition by Scribe Design, Gillingham, Kent
Originated, printed and bound in Singapore by
Toppan Printing Company (S) Pte Ltd

Contents

Acknowledgments

This book would not have been possible without the encouragement and generosity of my colleagues. I am grateful to the many fine clinicians who have supplied me with visual material, and I have recorded my acknowledgment under the appropriate captions. The publishers of *Dental Update* and *Restorative Dentistry* have graciously given permission to reproduce several figures.

Dr David Brown and Professor Michael Braden provided much valuable assistance in matters relating to materials science. Special help was given by Drs Osama Atta, David Auger, Chong Lin Chew, Andrew Flood, Charles Hopkins, Edward Lynch, Professor Keith Mortimer, Drs John Nasedkin, Simon Northeast, Dayananda Samarawickrama, Bernard Smith, Alastair Stokes, Brian Williams and Michael Wise. Professor Harry Allred gave me his support and encouragement throughout.

Allen Grey and Michael Kelly were most generous with their expertise in providing some of the scanning electron micrographs. In the dental laboratory the skills of Larry Browne, Michael Cattell, Malcolm Gill, Anthony Laurie and Tony Riseley were invaluable.

The line-drawings were made by Debbie Fenton and Ling Kemp. Their individual artistic abilities are much appreciated.

I am grateful to Martin Dunitz Limited for giving me the opportunity to write this book, and in particular to Mary Banks and her editorial team for their efficiency and forbearance. Especial thanks are due to Robert Peden and Jane Sugarman for their astute and sympathetic editing.

Whilst in the throes of writing this book, I was often reminded of two sayings by latter-day writers: 'Writing is easy; all you do is sit staring at a blank sheet of paper until the drops of blood form on your forehead' (Gene Fowler); and 'What no wife of a writer can ever understand is that a writer is working when he's staring out of the window' (Burton Rascoe). Thus to my long-suffering wife I offer my heartfelt gratitude for her patience and understanding.

WMT

Preface

Minimalism, a concept that is usually the province of the arts and social sciences, is now much discussed among the ranks of restorative dentists. One often hears of 'minimal preparations' or, indeed, 'non-preparations' in the description of such procedures as fillings and bridges. This mood of conservatism has arisen partly out of altruistic concern for the welfare of our patients and partly from a greater understanding of dental disease processes and the biophysical factors that may influence the effectiveness of the restorations we place in our patients' mouths. From the patient's point of view the benefits from these developments are obvious—less discomfort is experienced, and dental treatment is less arduous and fear-ridden.

It is now a cliché to say that the acid-etch technique has revolutionized restorative dentistry. Most dentists know about it; dental students are introduced to it even before they enter the clinical domains. Resin-bonded bridgework is an obvious extension of this technique, bringing with it a simplicity of concept and execution that attracts the 'average' practitioner who would otherwise shy away from the so-called 'conventional' bridgework which demands training and expertise. But therein lies the nub of the problem, for simplicity often encourages carelessness, overconfidence and complacency.

Therefore, although this book is about resin-bonded bridges, I trust there are sufficient pointers throughout the text to remind the informed reader that the basic principles of bridgework hold true. Indeed, success can only be derived from sound clinical judgement nurtured by many years of practical experience. Resin-bonded bridgework began almost as a clinical novelty. There were remarkable successes and stupendous failures. But a growing band of enthusiasts around the world, willing to share their findings in dental conferences and scientific publications, has led to the technique being accepted as a viable one. This book is both a compilation of that pool of knowledge and a pointer to future developments that will occur if the technique is to progress and remain an essential element in the care of our patients. The numerous citations in the text and the extensive list of references at the end of the book attest to the continuing research in this field.

F.W. Craddock in his book on *Dental Writing* defines a Preface as 'that part of a book in which an author may anticipate his critics'. Thus, I have placed the 'why' and the 'how' of resin-bonded bridges in the last two chapters of the book rather than at the beginning as is the custom with most textbooks on crowns and bridges. Instead, I have chosen to tell the story of resin-bonded bridges from the beginning, tracing their development to the present forms. There then follow two chapters on bonding methods and materials, to emphasize the need for good adhesion of bridge to tooth to ensure success. A chapter on resin-bonded bridge design and how it differs from that of conventional bridges precedes the final chapter on clinical procedures, which contains a collection of useful hints and tips—my own and those passed on by helpful colleagues. It may dismay some readers to find a fairly extensive section on bridge failures, but the well-known maxim that we all learn from our mistakes is aptly suited to this situation, and much current practice is based on this learning experience.

I have written this book with practitioners, technicians and students in mind, but I trust there is sufficient matter to interest research workers as well, for in the words of Michael Buonocore, the father of the acid-etch technique: 'Methodology without rationale is like memory without understanding.'

1 Types of resin-bonded bridges

Simple vanity makes most of us desire a perfect set of teeth. For people in Westernized societies this means that teeth deformed or ravaged by dental disease need to be restored to their natural colour and form. Even for the Ancient Greeks and Phoenicians, it was probably vanity rather than the wish to chew better that kept their craftsmen busy producing false teeth.

Naturally, considerable advances have been made since those times, but aesthetic dentistry still depends on the replacement and simulation of the hard and soft tissues of the mouth. It was the introduction of acrylic polymers in 1937 that gave dentists the means to do this cheaply and easily. Acrylic resins, suitably tinted and moulded, may mimic the appearance of gums and teeth in a way no other material can. Improvements in manufacturing techniques have resulted in a remarkable degree of sophistication, whereby colour may be incorporated in layers and a realistic characterization achieved. But as far as artificial teeth are concerned, the full porcelain veneer crown must be regarded as the ultimate in aesthetic restoration. The skill and dedication of the expert technician in producing a porcelain crown may be equated to that of a master ceramist creating a work of art (Figure 1.1).

Among the innovations that have changed the practice of dentistry over the last two decades, the acid-etch technique and the use of composite resins can be regarded as some of the most influential. In 1955 M. Buonocore, a researcher at the Eastman Dental Center in Rochester, New York, made the astute observation that the application

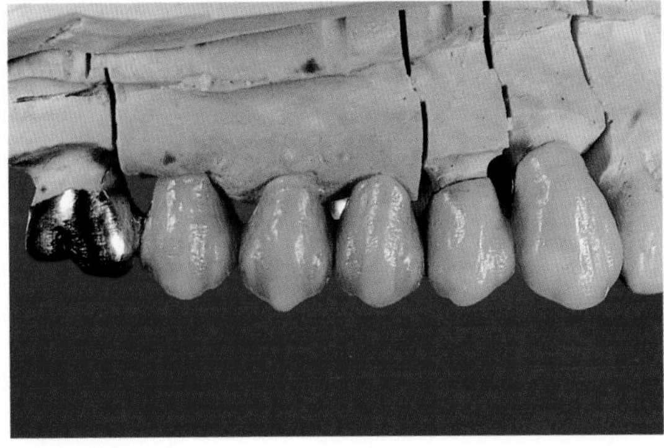

a

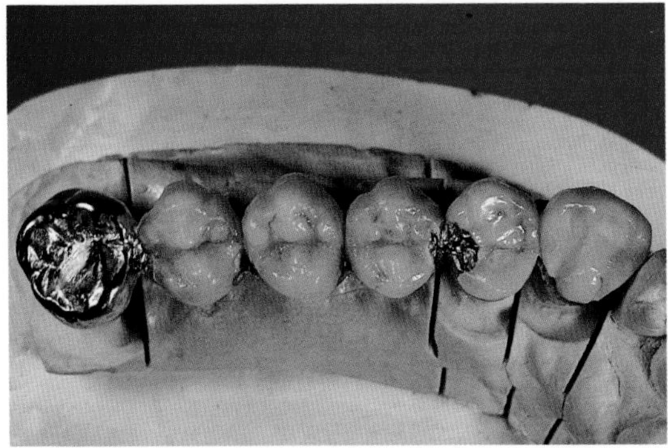

b

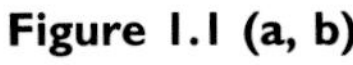

Figure 1.1 (a, b)

An example of the dental ceramist's skill in reproducing tooth colour and form. (Technician: Mr E. Barden.)

of a weak inorganic acid could alter the surface of enamel such that bonding of a resin to the surface could take place. Buonocore experimented with acrylic resins but found these were much too weak to withstand the stresses exerted upon them in the mouth. It was not until R. Bowen (1963) developed a unique system containing 25 per cent by weight of a polymerizable monomer and 75 per cent by weight of a vitreous filler—the composite resin—that the acid-etch technique could become an effective procedure.

The usual method of producing crowns and bridges is by bulk reduction of the crowns of teeth using cutting burs to create sufficient space for a veneer of metal and/or porcelain. The procedure is time-consuming, exacting, often uncomfortable for the patient and expensive. For some patients, especially the very young and the very old, the experience can be rather exhausting due to the extensive dental sessions. In young teeth with large pulps, tooth preparation may even be hazardous. Thus, a technique which involves very little tooth tissue removal and obviates the need for local anaesthetics, and which allows the practitioner simply to 'stick on' a false tooth to bridge an edentulous gap, would have many attractions. These bridges may be simple, single units directly attached to the abutment teeth, or complex, multiunit designs often incorporating precision attachments. The common denominator in all cases is the composite resin 'adhesive' between the bridge and the etched tooth surface.

For convenience, the resin-bonded bridges may be classified according to the manner in which the replacement tooth, or pontic, is attached (bonded) to the adjacent tooth surfaces (Box A). These are either *direct-bonded* at the chairside, usually as an 'emergency' procedure, or *indirect-bonded* via prefabricated attachments or frameworks constructed and prepared in the laboratory. This classification is by no means final. As with any innovative technique, continual changes are being incorporated as more knowledge and clinical expertise are gained and tougher resins with greater adhesive power are developed. Indeed, the classification in itself reflects the evolution in design of the resin-bonded bridge.

Direct-bonded attachments

The natural tooth as the pontic

This usually occurs either in a traumatized incisor where the root has been so severely fractured that reimplantation is not feasible or the tooth may have suffered irreversible bone loss from periodontal disease, becoming very loose as a consequence (Posner, 1985). In each case, the root is trimmed to within a few millimetres below the amelocemental junction. Pulp remnants are removed and the root canal cleaned thoroughly; it is then filled with amalgam at the apical one-third and with composite resin in the coronal access cavity. The treated tooth is then bonded to the etched approximal surfaces of the abutment teeth using a suitable composite resin (Figure 1.2).

Resin tooth pontics

It is also possible to construct a pontic from an acrylic or, indeed, a composite resin using a cellulose acetate or polycarbonate crown form as a mould. Alternatively, stock acrylic denture teeth may be used. The pontic is trimmed at the chairside or laboratory before being bonded to the abutment teeth (Figure 1.3).

The main advantage of direct-bonded teeth or pontics is convenience because only one visit is usually necessary. However, there is a tendency for the composite bond to break under stress (Figure 1.4), although the joints may be reinforced by accessory retention, eg undercutting, mesh strips (Figure 1.5; see also Figure 1.2c–f), threaded pins and stainless steel wire. Nevertheless difficulty in achieving good aesthetics and embrasure form (which is also necessary for effective oral hygiene) has resulted in alternative methods being devised.

Indirect-bonded bridges

Orthodontic brackets/pads

By carrying the pontic on a metal subframe and then bonding the frame to the etched teeth using a thin film of composite resin as a 'cement', occurrence of cohesive bond fractures is reduced. The simplest method is to use the orthodontic brackets or pads common in fixed appliance therapy (Fleming, 1981; Jones and Richards, 1984). These brackets, which present a regular pitted pattern on the surface to be fitted, ie the fit surface, enable firm retention of the composite resin to the etched enamel surface. The pads may be adapted to the lingual or approximal surfaces of acrylic or porcelain pontics.

Lingual pads

The framework may be made of two or more preformed orthodontic pads which are electrically welded to a connecting stainless steel wire of rectangular cross-section; this, in turn, supports the pontic anchored in a retention slot on the lingual surface with acrylic resin that is cured at room temperature (Figure 1.6). It is important that the wire is accurately bent to lie passively on the lingual surfaces of the abutment teeth. Any inadvertent distortion in the wire could cause an embarrassing 'orthodontic effect'.

Approximal pads

Here again, the pontics may be stock acrylic or porcelain teeth. It is possible to use either photo-etched stainless steel pads or polycarbonate brackets and these are retained with acrylic resin within slots in the approximal surfaces of the pontic (Figure 1.7). This technique is sometimes known as the FABB (Fleming acrylic-composite bonded bridge) technique after its designer (Fleming, 1981).

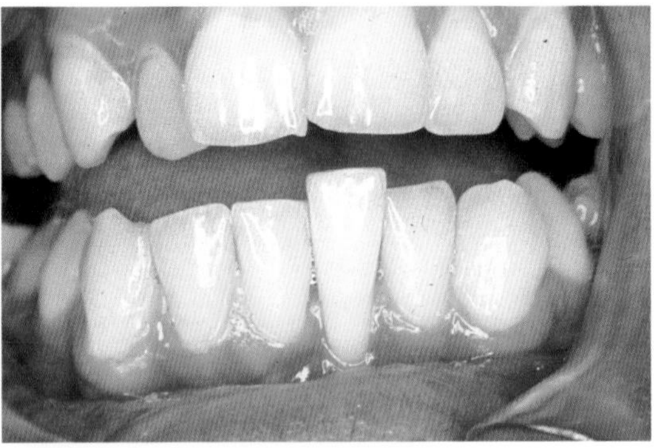

Figure 1.2

(a) Periodontal disease has affected the lower left central incisor, and gross irreversible bone loss has resulted in mobility and extrusion of the tooth.

(b) The dental radiograph shows the extent of bone loss.

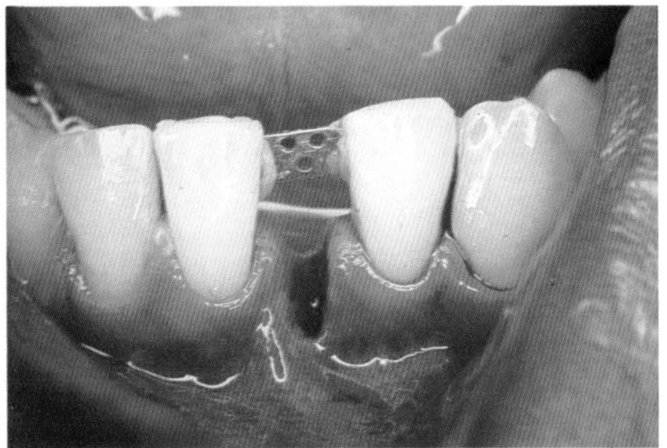

(c) Extraction of the tooth has been carried out, and a malleable stainless steel perforated splint (Splint-Grid, Ellman) has been attached with composite resin to the etched lingual surfaces of the lower left lateral and right central incisors.

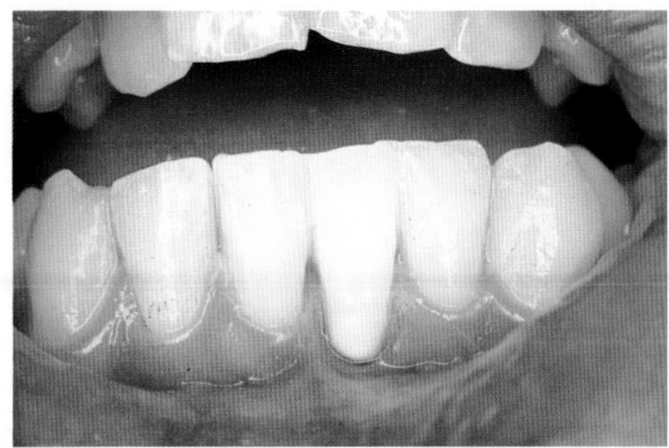

(d) The extracted tooth is cleaned and root-filled, and the root apex removed; the tooth is then reimplanted in the extraction socket and bonded to the splint.

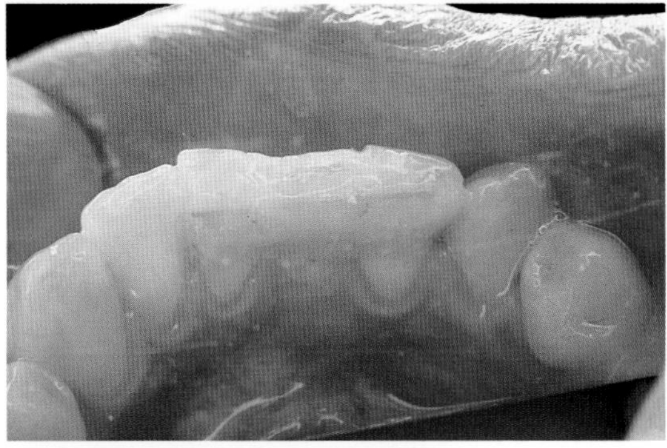

(e) Lingual view of the direct-bonded bridge.

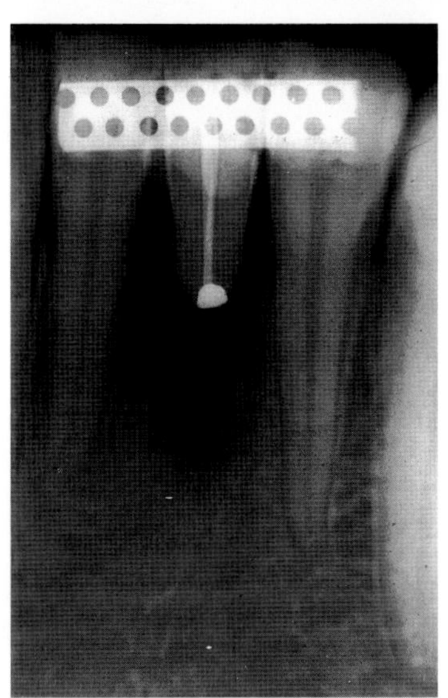

(f) Radiograph showing the splinted tooth in position. The amputated root is sealed at the apical aspect with a 'retrograde' amalgam filling. (Courtesy of Dr B.T. Posner.)

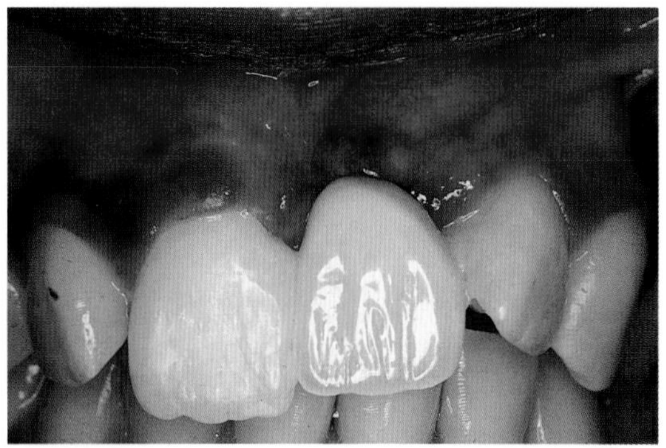
a

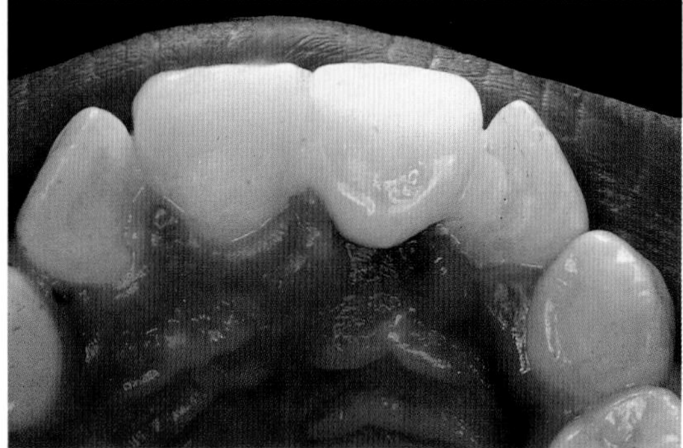
b

Figure 1.3 (a, b)

Direct-bonded resin tooth pontic replacing an upper left central incisor. Note the obliteration of the approximal embrasures to allow a reasonable thickness of composite resin for strength.

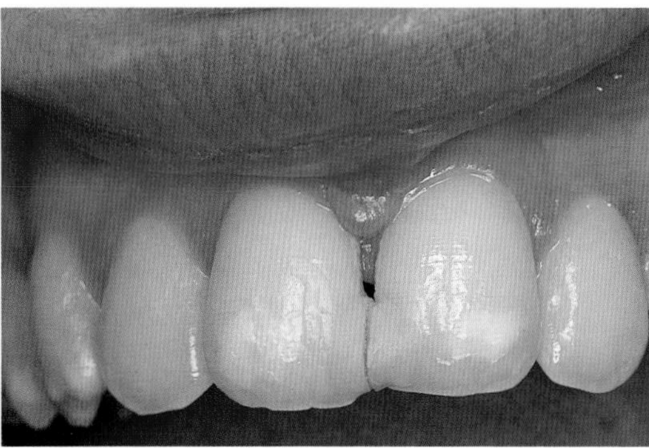

Figure 1.4

An inherent drawback of direct-bonded bridges is a tendency to fracture at the weakest area when subjected to biting stresses.

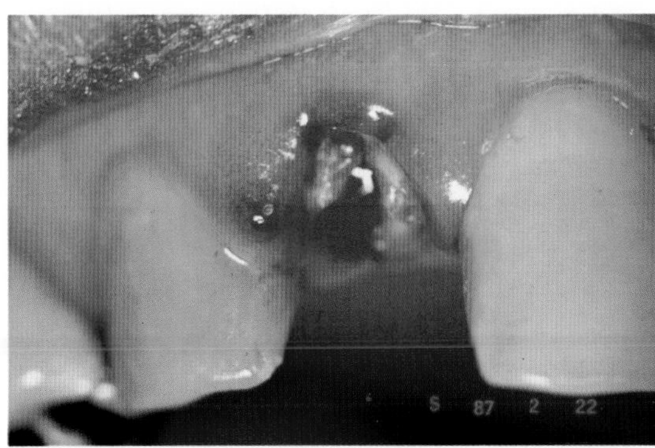

Figure 1.5

(a) Traumatized upper right lateral incisor in a young adult showing bleeding from the exposed pulp.

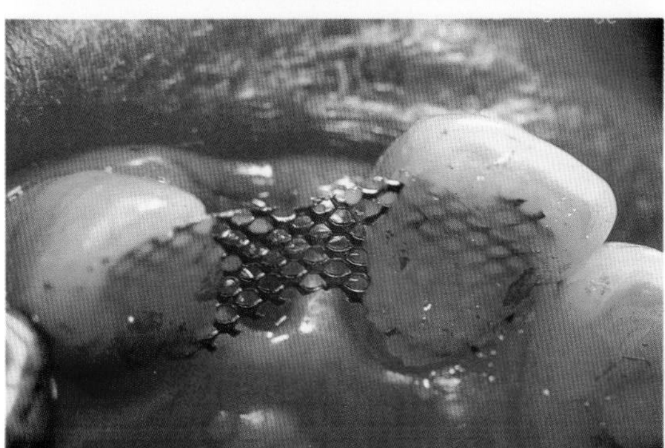

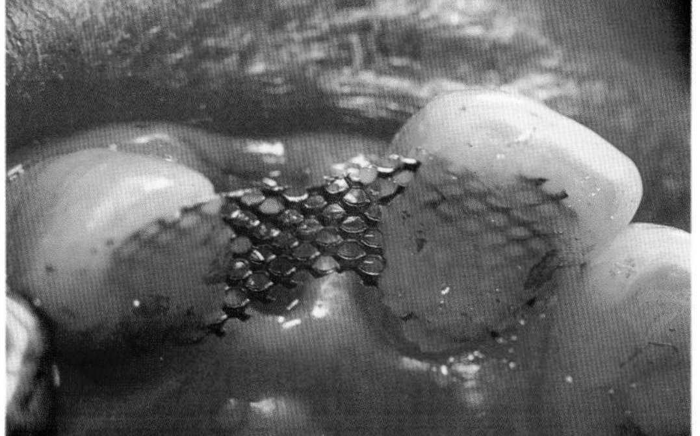

(b) The tooth has been extracted and a mesh splint attached to the abutment teeth with acid etching and composite resin.

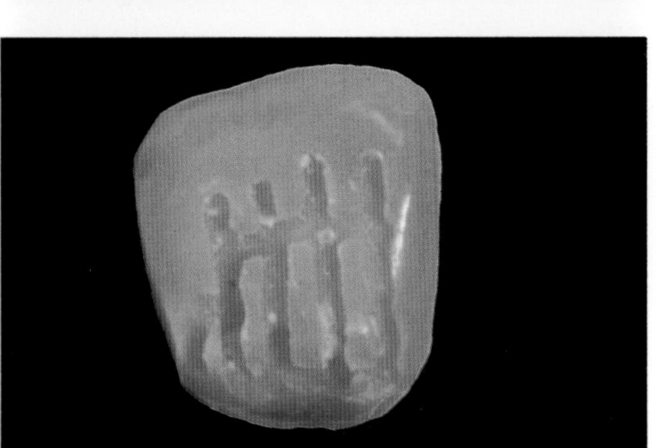

(c) Detail of the acrylic tooth to be used as a pontic, showing grooves to enhance retention to the composite resin.

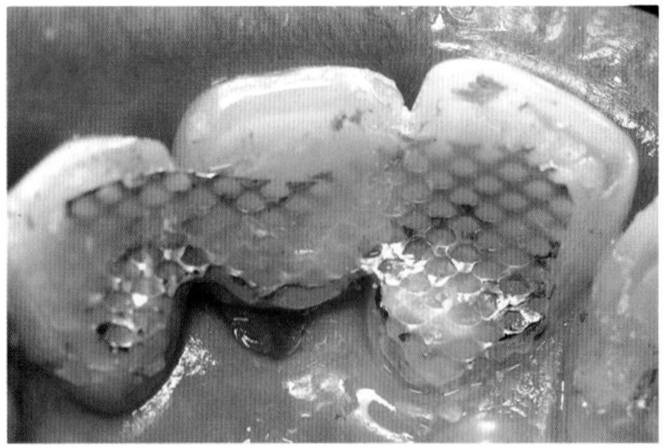

(d) The complete mesh-supported, direct-bonded bridge viewed from the lingual aspect.

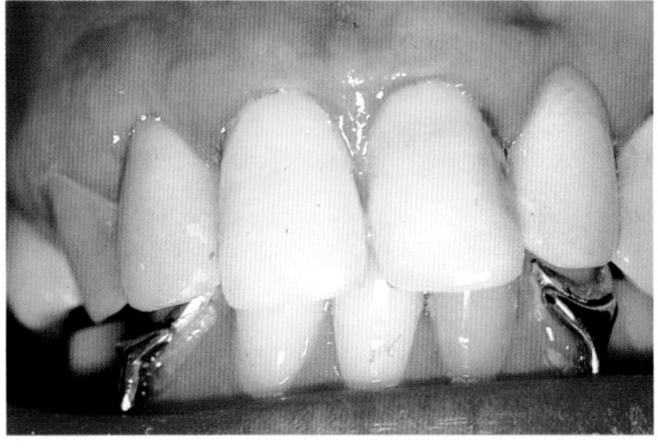

(e) The same from the labial aspect showing a satisfactory appearance but with inaccessible embrasures. (Courtesy of Dr S.E. Northeast.)

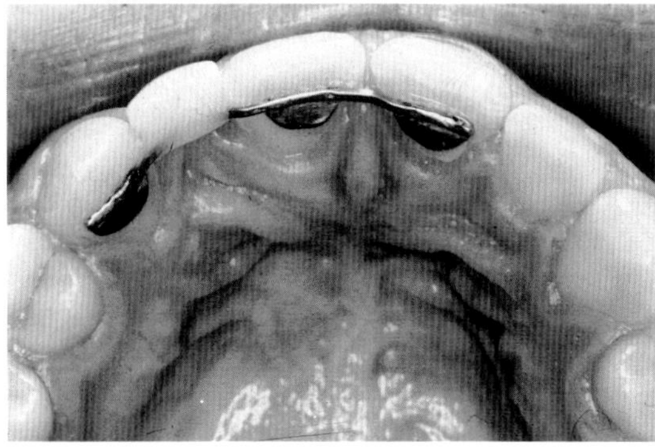

Figure 1.6

Acrylic pontic of an upper right lateral incisor supported on a stainless steel arch wire which is welded to three preformed stainless steel orthodontic pads. (Courtesy of Dr M.L. Jones.)

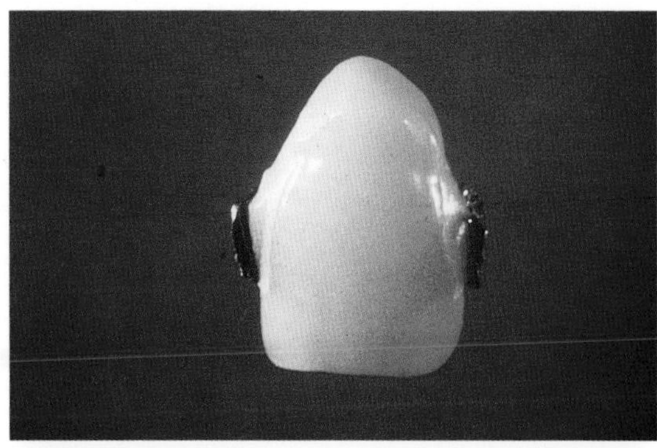

Figure 1.7

(a) FABB design—polycarbonate pontic with approximal stainless steel orthodontic pads.

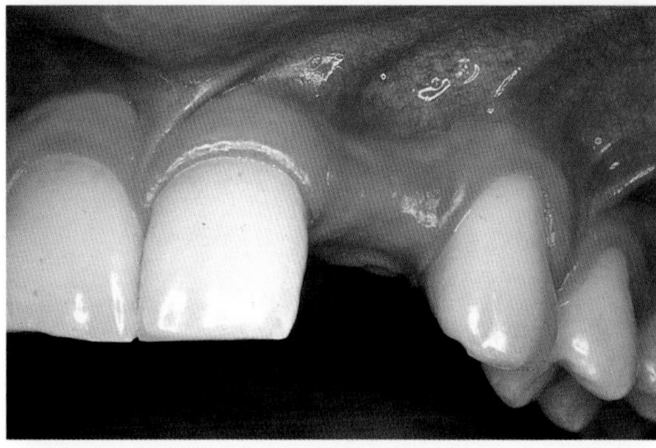

(b) Preoperative situation showing missing upper left lateral incisor.

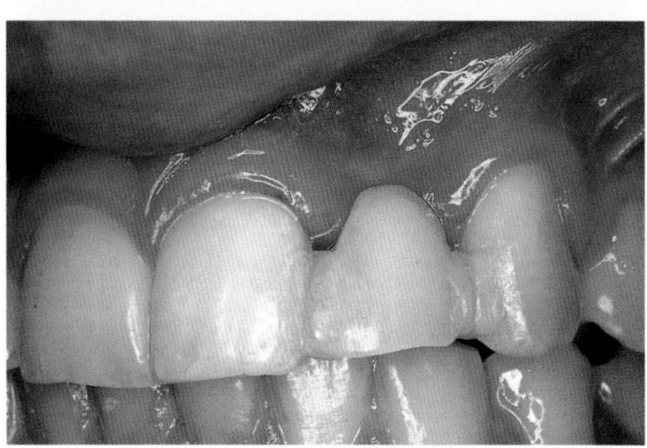

(c) Pontic bonded in place; note unsatisfactory embrasure form.

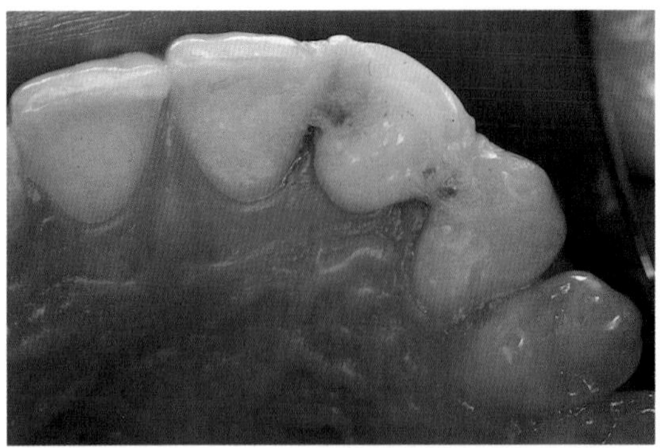

(d) Lingual aspect of the same.

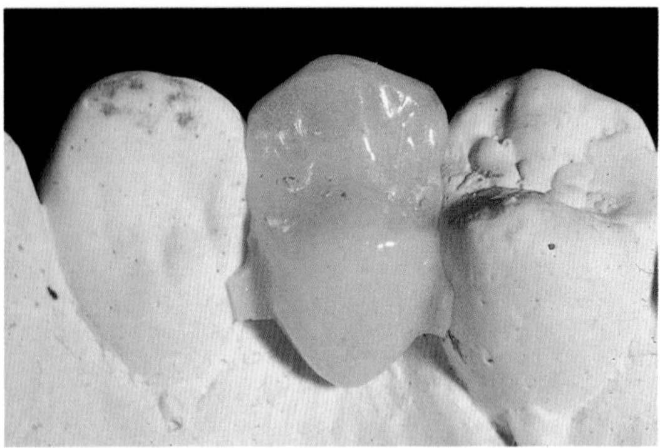

(e) Polycarbonate premolar pontic with polycarbonate orthodontic pads.

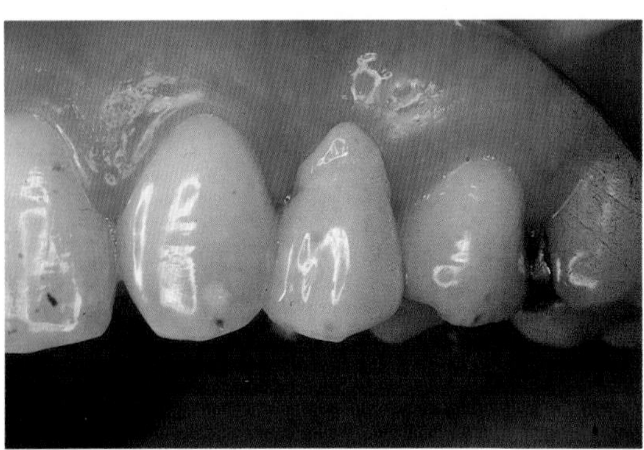

(f) The upper left first premolar pontic with approximal polycarbonate pads shows a more aesthetically acceptable embrasure form. (Courtesy of Dr H.B. Fleming.)

BOX A CLASSIFICATION OF RESIN-BONDED BRIDGES

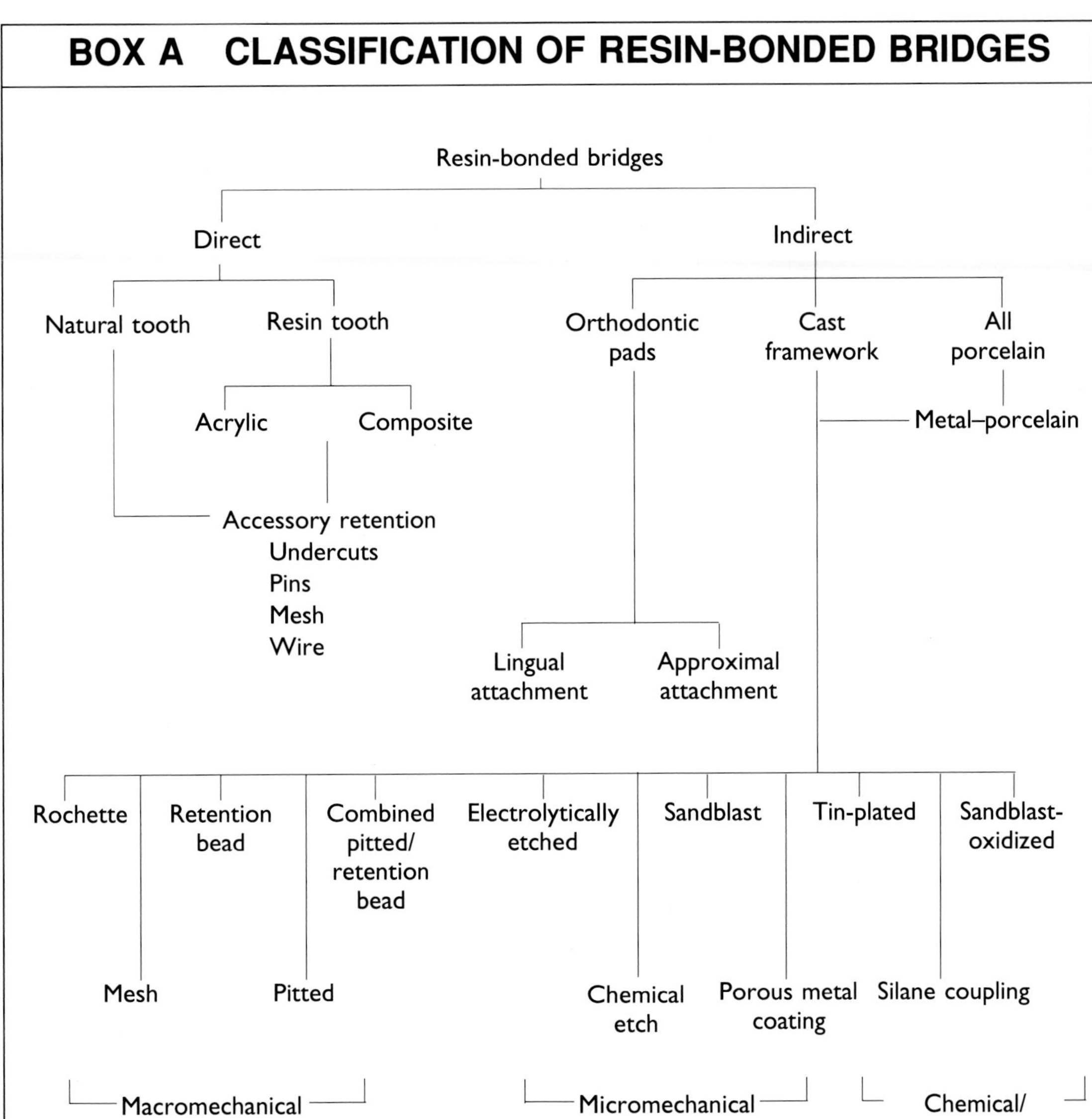

2 Cast metal framework

Metals may display resistance to bending (high stiffness) or breaking (high strength) in a unique way. Their distinctive atomic structure allows deformation in such a ductile manner and absorption of energy by such localized stretching that, under most conditions, any cracks in the structure cannot continue to the surface in the catastrophic way that is commonly seen in certain materials such as glass and porcelain.

These mechanical properties of high stiffness and strength enable metals to be used advantageously in dentistry where thin sections are often required. This is particularly important because, in the majority of designs for resin-bonded bridges, the retaining flanges are placed on, or may extend onto, the occlusal planes.

The metals used must also be able to resist tarnishing and corrosion in the moist environment of the mouth. Whilst a number of pure metals, such as gold, platinum, chromium and titanium, might resist the sort of chemical attack likely to be encountered in the mouth, the combination of their inherently poor mechanical properties, difficulty in being handled and high expense means that, in practice, mixtures of metals are employed—the dental alloys.

The third essential requirement for an alloy, as used in a resin-bonded bridge, is the capability of bonding to tooth tissue. Whereas etching of the tooth is now a well-established technique for creating an enamel surface that is attractive to resins, the creation of resin-to-metal bonds is fraught with difficulty. At present there are three basic ways of forming the resin-to-metal bond, and these are:

1 Cast-in mechanical features.
2 Specially developed mechanical features.
3 Surfaces capable of promoting or encouraging chemical bonding.

As is common in dentistry, some techniques can combine all three methods.

Cast-in mechanical features

Perforated (Rochette) design

Despite improvements in technique and materials, the early resin-bonded bridges were regarded more as a measure of exigency than a planned design for longevity. The first suggestion that this technique was feasible as a longer-term solution came from papers by A. Rochette (1972, 1973). He described a metal periodontal splint which was cast in one piece and which consisted of several perforated segments bonded to the etched lingual surfaces of teeth by composite resin (Figure 2.1). Any gaps in the dental arch which happened to be present could be easily filled in with a porcelain or acrylic pontic (Figures 2.2 and 2.3). This design is very popular in the United Kingdom and is often known by its eponym 'Rochette bridge'. Retention is solely by the mechanical locking of composite to the perforations in the metal flanges—the so-called *macromechanical mode* of retention. It does not seem to matter whether there are several small holes or one large hole, whether they are parallel-sided or countersunk (Figure 2.4), or whether indeed they have any sort of pattern—they all appear, at least in vitro, to provide sufficient retention against the dislodging forces that are probably encountered in the mouth (Williams et al, 1982; Saunders, 1984).

Drilling holes in the casting is both tedious and wasteful: a small rose head or dome-shaped tungsten carbide bur is used and, if the alloy is very hard, eg cobalt–chromium, several burs may have to be used.

Alternatively, the perforations can be incorporated into the wax pattern itself. The framework is waxed up on the working casts often with the flange less than 0.7 mm thick and with a thin bevelled margin. Holes are sunk in the wax pattern

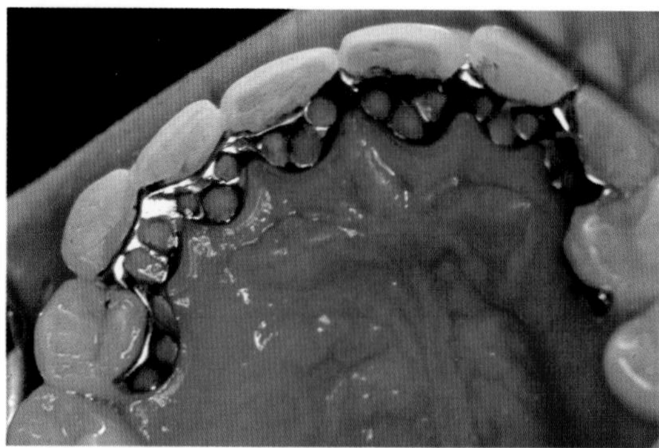

Figure 2.1

Perforated metal splint based on the Rochette design.

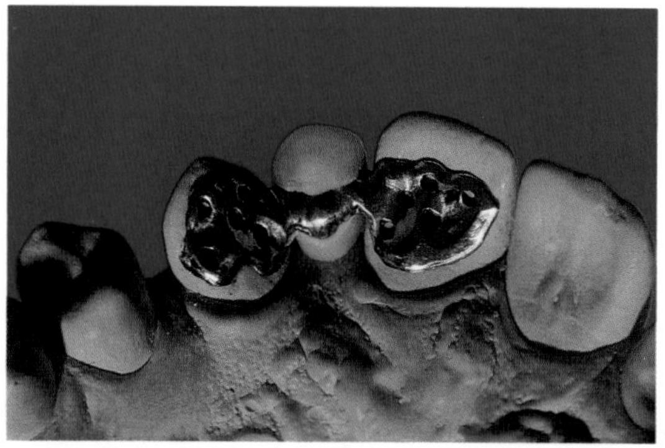

a

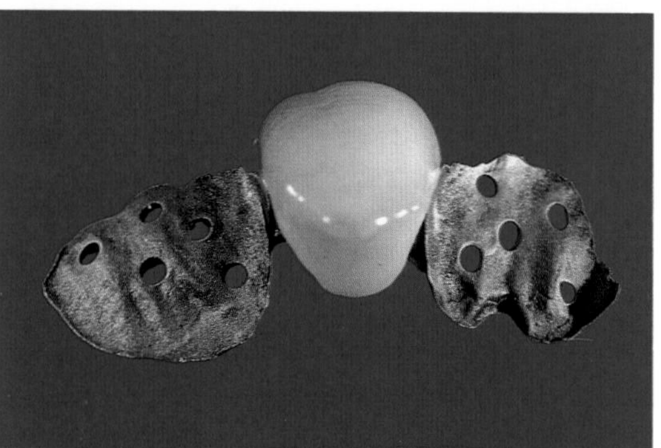

b

Figure 2.2 (a, b)

Rochette bridge showing perforated metal flanges and porcelain pontic. The alloy used had a semi-precious content.

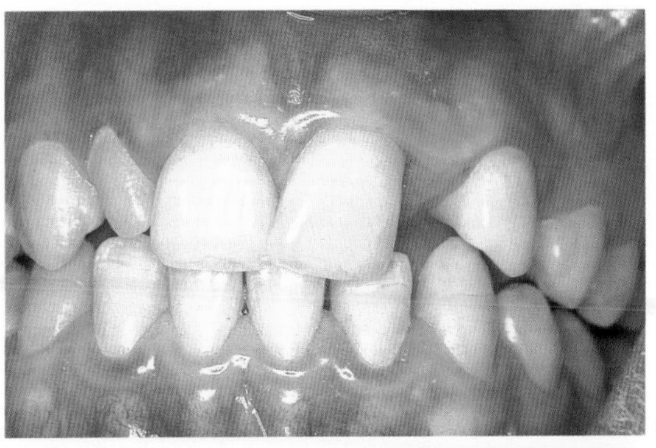

a

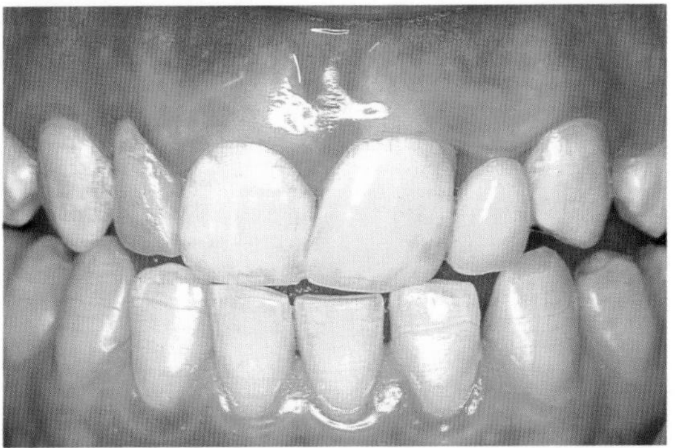

b

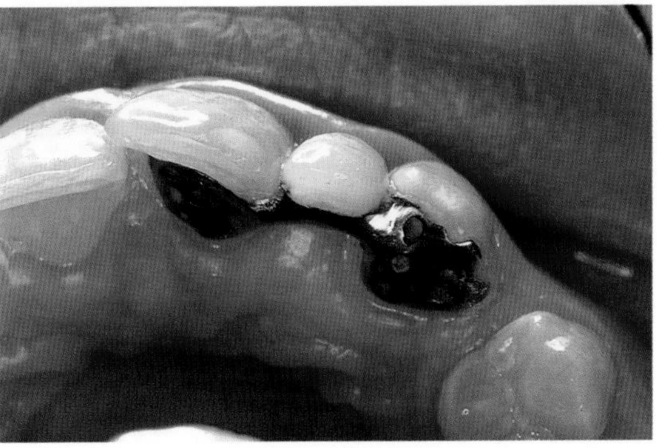

c

Figure 2.3

(a) Preoperative situation with missing upper left lateral incisor.

(b, c) Completed Rochette bridge bonded in place with microfilled composite resin, after acid etching of the abutment teeth.

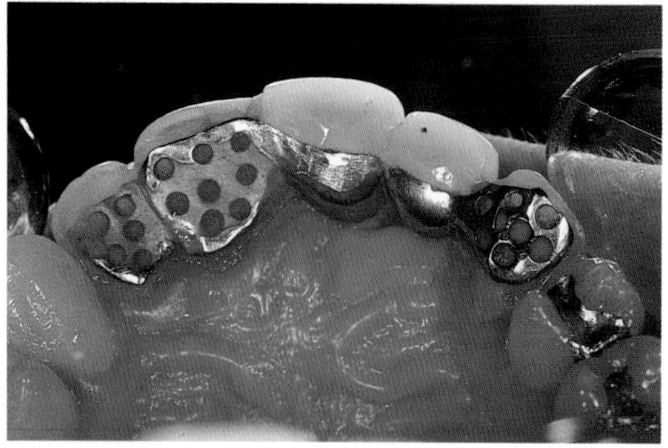

Figure 2.4

Variations in the number and size of perforations may not affect the retention of the bridge but may result in a weakening of the flange, as in the upper left canine. Note excess resin has covered the surface of the flange on the upper right lateral and central incisor flanges.

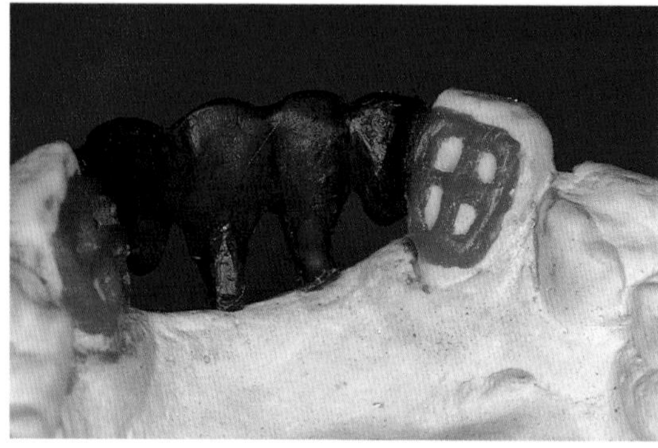

Figure 2.5

Rochette bridge with window-frame pattern made from preformed wax rods.

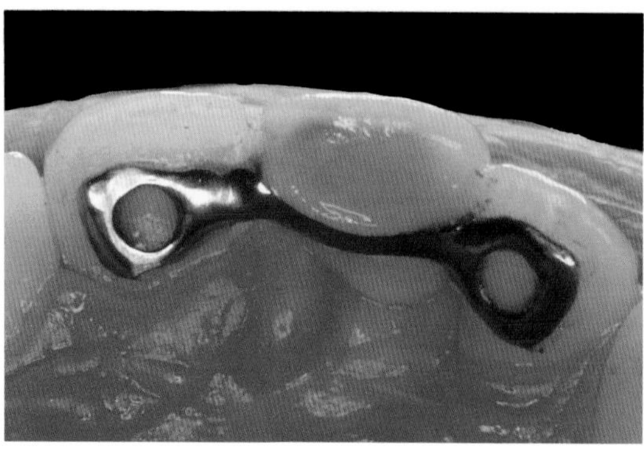

Figure 2.6

Rochette bridge—single-hole 'fishmouth' design. (Courtesy of Dr R. Boggia.)

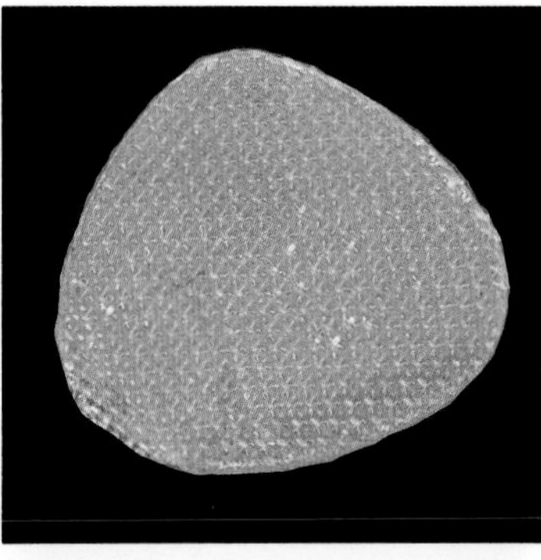

Figure 2.7

Duralingual (Unitek Corp.) polyester mesh pattern.

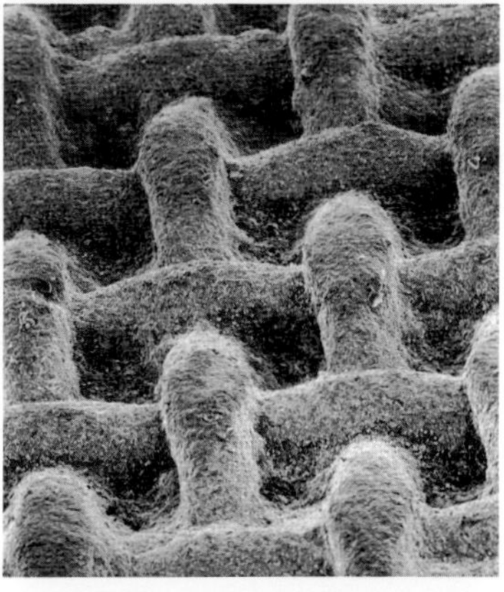

Figure 2.8

Scanning electron micrograph (SEM) of a cast-in surface created in a nickel–chromium alloy from: (a) Duralingual (Unitek Corp.) mesh.

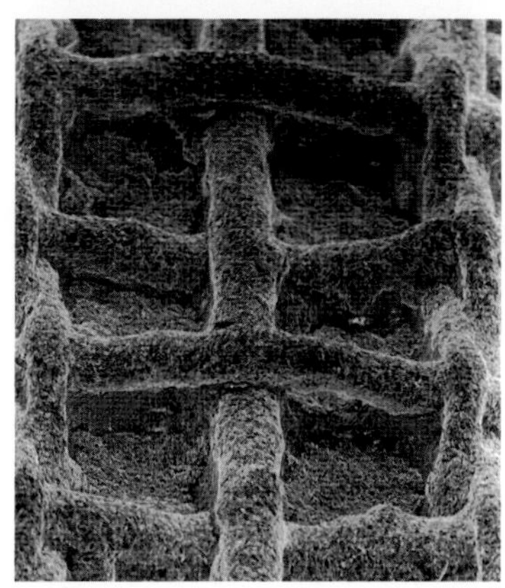

(b) Klett-o-Bond (Renfert) mesh. (Magnification x 203.) (Courtesy of Dr O. Atta.)

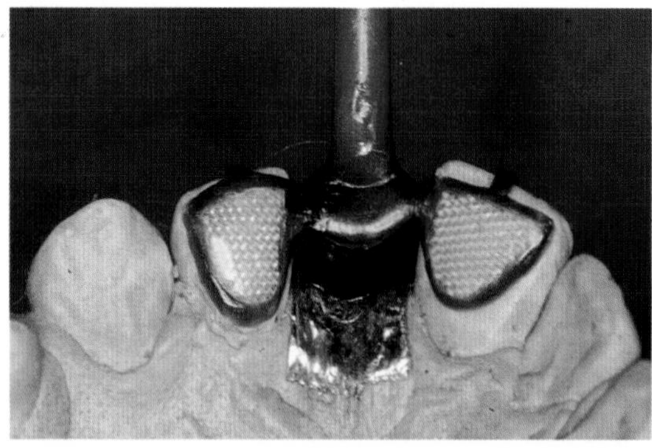

Figure 2.9

Wax-up of a bridge using the Duralingual mesh.

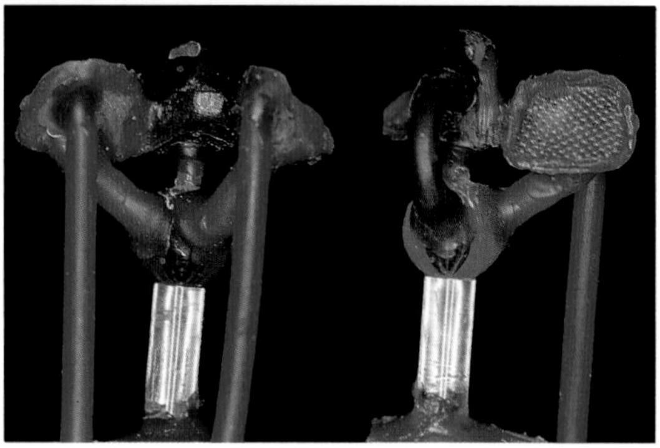

Figure 2.10

Additional venting sprues must be incorporated to prevent voids in the casting.

with a heated probe, and may be countersunk with a heated ball-ended burnisher.

Preformed wax rods may also be used to produce a sort of window-frame pattern (Figure 2.5) or an open 'fishmouth' design (Figure 2.6). As mentioned before, provided results of in vitro tests are valid, almost any pattern is suitable so long as it provides good mechanical retention of the resin on the metal surface.

Mesh pattern flange

This technique employs a polyester or nylon mesh backed up with a veneer of wax to produce the pattern which is cast in a dental alloy. The original concept arose from use of pieces cut out of a domestic, nylon mesh sieve and set within the wax pattern; these would burn out leaving an imprint of the mesh in the casting. Two commercial kits are available: Duralingual (Unitek) and Klett-o-Bond (Renfert). Both consist of several different wing shapes of polyester or nylon mesh backed by a veneer of wax (Figure 2.7). They differ in the size of the weave, with Klett-o-Bond having the larger size (Figure 2.8).

A suitable pattern is selected and trimmed to fit approximately to an outline pencilled on the cast. The mesh side is placed towards the lingual surface of the abutment tooth. The rough edges of the mesh must be sealed with inlay wax, preferably using an electric wax knife to avoid overheating as this could cause the wax to smear the mesh structure; the margins are then bevelled (Figure 2.9).

Owing to the intricacies of the mesh pattern, miscasts are quite common when conventional spruing techniques are used. To avoid the formation of voids in the casting, additional venting sprues should be incorporated, particularly from the most extreme margin of the pattern to the outer rim (Figure 2.10). The application of a

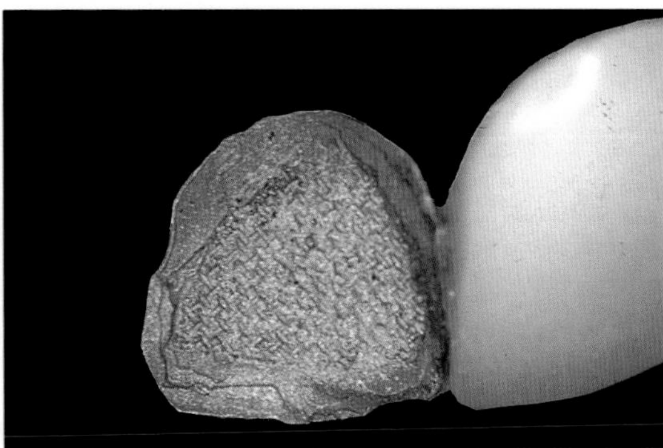

Figure 2.11

(a) Casting of Duralingual mesh. Note large area of margin with no mesh pattern.

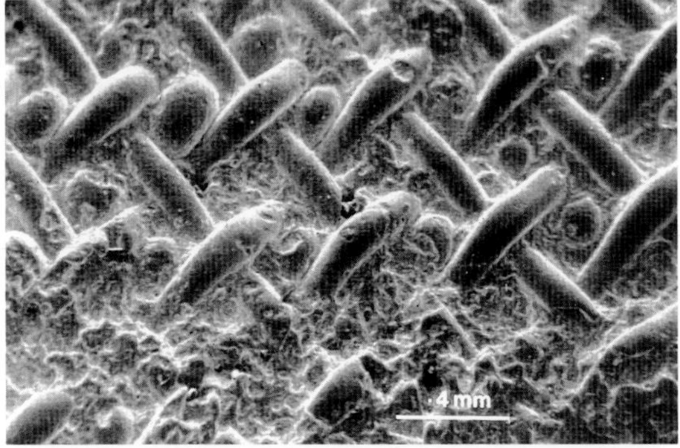

(b) SEM of the same showing miscast area. The fine weave of the mesh is believed to cause this problem.

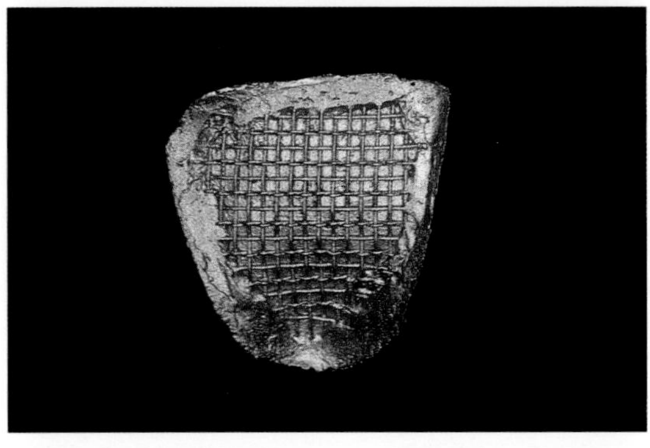

Figure 2.12

(a) Casting of Klett-o-Bond mesh.

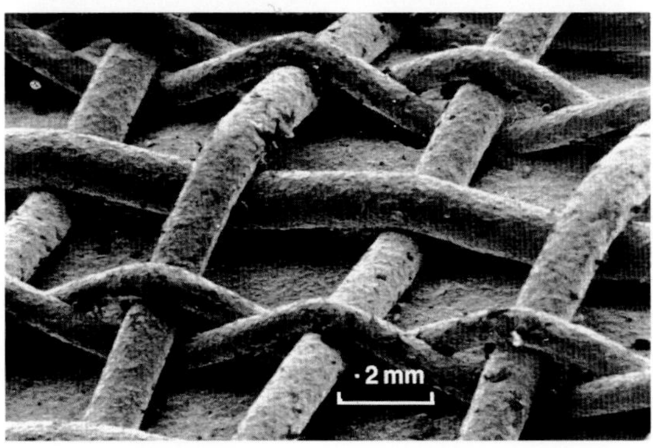

(b) SEM. The coarser weave of the pattern reduces the chances of a miscast and enhances retention of the resin.

wetting agent to the wax pattern before investing also assists in a reduction in the casting defects.

The magnified image of the casting (Figures 2.11 and 2.12) demonstrates the mechanical retention afforded by this system, which can be verified by viewing through a hand lens or a low power microscope. The difficulty in obtaining a perfect cast of the fine interweaving pattern (Figure 2.11) is also evident, although the broader weave pattern (Figure 2.12) tends to produce a better cast. It is claimed (Taleghani et al, 1987) that the retention of composite resin by the mesh is as strong as the retention on an etched metal surface (see below), although the need to seal the mesh at the margins may leave large areas with no mechanical retention (Figures 2.11a and 2.12a).

Particle-roughened flange

Resin retention to metal surfaces may be achieved by incorporating retention beads, which form a pitted pattern, or by combining pits with beads.

Retention beads are available in the form of acrylic resin (LaBarre and Ward, 1984) or other calcinable material (Wiltshire and Ferreira, 1987) which will burn out in the casting process.

A pitted surface on a cast metal flange may be achieved by embedding common salt grains 0.15–0.25 mm in size (using standard sieves) in a matrix of inlay resin or wax (Figure 2.13). On immersion of the pattern in water, the salt grains dissolve away leaving sharp depressions or pits which are reproduced in the casting (Figure 2.14). This is sometimes known as the *Virginia salt*

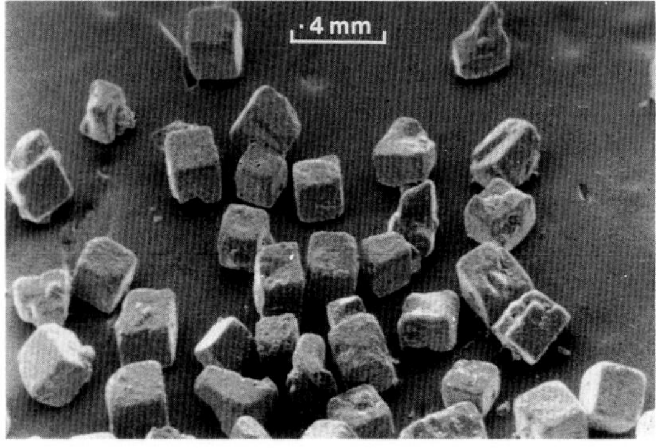

Figure 2.13

SEM of common salt grains used in creating a pitted surface.

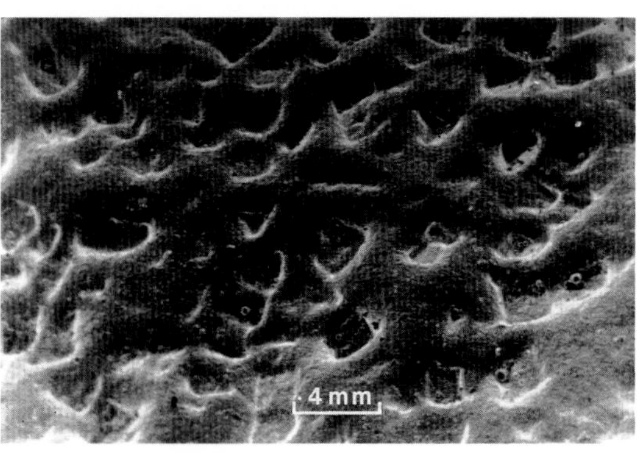

Figure 2.14

SEM of casting showing depressions left by the salt grains.

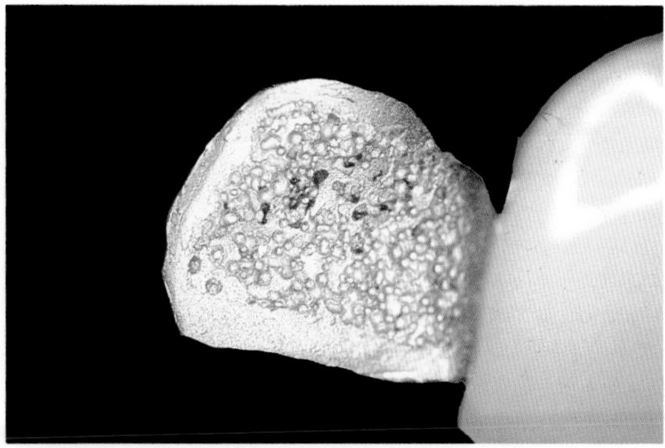

Figure 2.15

(a) The surface of fit of a Crystal Bond casting, showing again the large area of margin devoid of retention.

(b) SEM of the same (magnification x 101.5) showing retentive pits and beads.

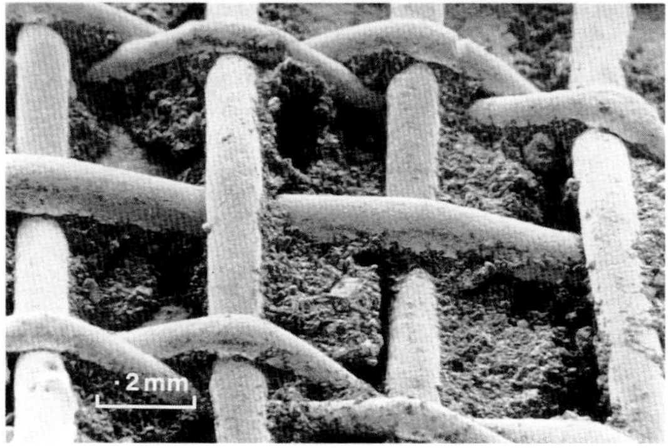

Figure 2.16

Where there is little undercut in cast-in mechanical features, the resin cement is likely to come apart.

technique or the *Virginia bridge* because of its origins in the Medical College of Virginia in Richmond, Virginia, USA (Hudgins et al, 1985; Moon, 1987). A commercial product (Crystal Bond) employing this idea, but also incorporating fine acrylic beads for extra retention, is available (combined pitted/beaded pattern).

The technique of applying the beads and/or salt grains is very simple. A water-soluble adhesive gel is first painted onto the outlined flange area on the dry stone cast. The grains and/or beads are dusted over the painted area, pressed gently in place and the excess shaken off. After allowing a few minutes for the adhesive to dry, inlay wax or resin is then applied into and around the flange area. The remainder of the bridge components is completed in the usual manner and the wax-up sprued for investing. The complete wax pattern is released from the cast by immersion in a basin of water at room temperature. Further gentle rinsing with cold water is necessary to dissolve all the soluble salt grains if these are used. The pattern is then invested and cast.

The pitted–beaded surface of a casting is seen in Figure 2.15. The 'pits' and 'beads' can be viewed under low-power magnification, and provide *macromechanical* retention for the composite resin. But again, as with the mesh technique, the margins are often left without a visibly retentive surface.

Limitations of the cast-in (macromechanical) surface

In practice, the ability of resins to bond to macromechanical retentive surfaces depends as much on the 'retentiveness' of the pattern as on what happens to the bond during stress loading.

If loaded in a 'tensile' manner, ie with a pulling force, fracture of the weakest sections of the structural features may occur. It is more probable, however, that the resin will be pulled out of those simple features that have little in the way of an undercut (Figure 2.16). In heavily undercut areas, the resin is likely to fracture 'in tension'.

If loaded with a shearing force, probably only the resin will fail, and there would be little 'pull-out' occurring *unless* the resin was excessively 'elastic'. The greater the number of retentive resin-to-metal links, the stronger the bond.

In the case of the Rochette bridge, there is macroscopic retention and the bond strength is influenced by the total cross-sectional area of the resin at the smallest hole diameter. Thus, as mentioned previously, it does not matter whether there is a solitary hole or several small holes in the retainer, the actual number usually being governed by convenience and practicality. Retention is confined to the immediate region of the perforation, which effectively concentrates occlusal stresses on the few narrow protrusions of resin. If failure occurs, it does so at the isthmus of the resin. Furthermore, exposed resin at the perforations could be subjected to abrasion or microleakage (Figure 2.17).

In a similar fashion, the perforations in Rochette flanges invariably weaken the bridge (Figure 2.18) and, in compensation, the flanges are often thickened, in turn creating occlusal interferences. The inference from this is that a non-perforated design (Figure 2.19) would enhance the durability of the restoration by protecting the resin.

In other examples of cast-in retention, the total area available for potential bonding is high, but resistance to tensile dislodging forces can only develop if the resin is able to flow into undercut areas.

Another problem concerns the resin itself. Often there is a mismatch in the coefficients of thermal expansion of resin and metal; coupled with the innate polymerization shrinkage of resins, the result could be a separation of the two components.

Specially developed mechanical features

Etched metal

Buonocore drew his inspiration for the acid-etch technique from industry, where phosphoric acid preparations were routinely used to treat metal surfaces to achieve greater adhesion of paint and resin coatings. In a similar manner, McLaughlin (1981) in New York, and Thompson and associates at the University of Maryland (1981), derived the etched metal technique from the well-known phenomenon found in corrosion engineering called 'pitting'. Controlled pitting corrosion or etching of metal is achieved by electrochemical or

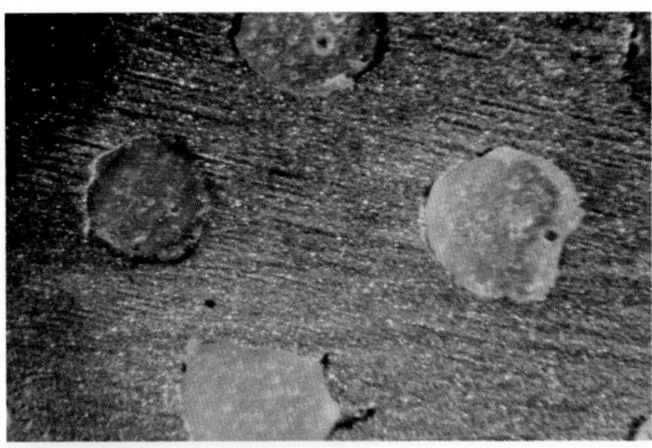

Figure 2.17

(a) The fit (inner) surface of a Rochette type flange after fracture of the resin showing the resin only within the retentive holes. (Courtesy of Dr D. Brown.).

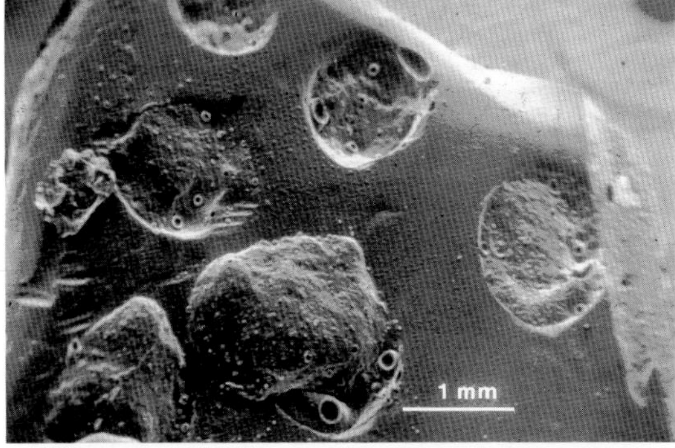

(b) SEM of the outer surface showing different degrees of wear affecting the resin.

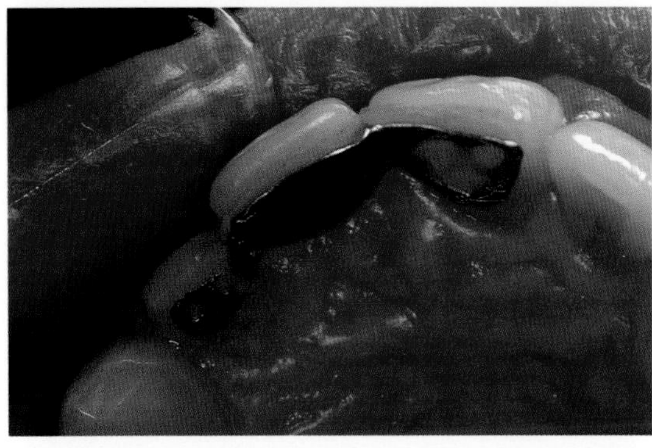

Figure 2.18

Fractured flange weakened by large perforations.

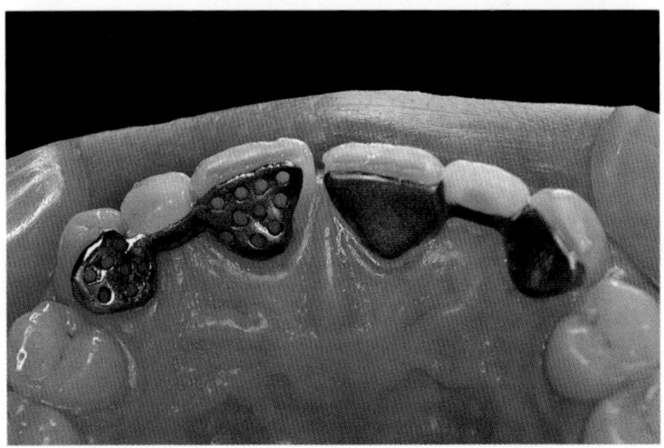

Figure 2.19

Left: perforated Rochette design; right: non-perforated design.

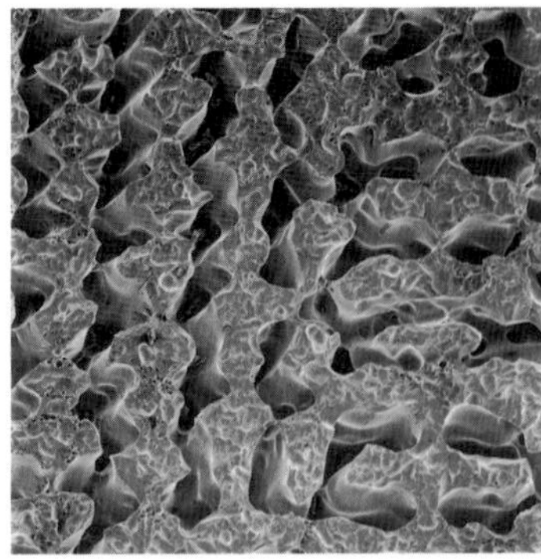

Figure 2.20

(a) SEM of electrolytically etched alloy, NP2. (Magnification × 812.)

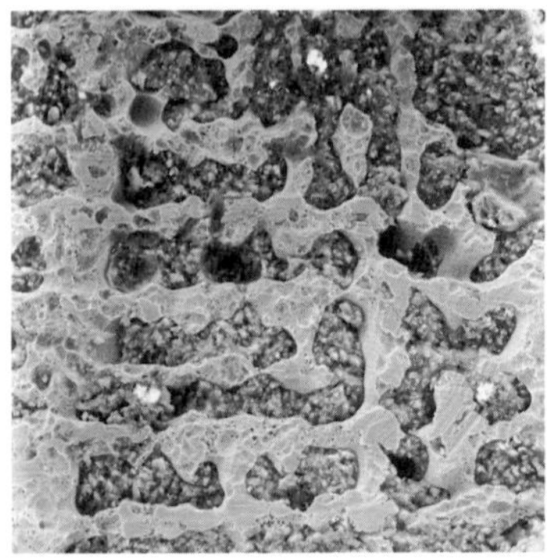

(b) The same, showing resin retained within the pores of the etched metal. Resin (Comspan) was fractured off during tensile testing. (Courtesy of Dr O. Atta.)

chemical means, and is usually applied to special dental alloys to produce effective pitted and porous patterns on the metal surface, such as the pattern seen in Figure 2.20a. The composite resin becomes attached (albeit mainly mechanically) through the permeation of the fine ramifications of the etched metal surface (Figure 2.20b)—a 'micromechanical mode' of retention. The Maryland (or McLaughlin) bridge (as it is known) is now well established as a prevalent resin-bonded bridge, especially in the USA.

Different etch patterns may be produced according to the composition and (in metallurgical terms) the 'dendritic structure' of the alloys (Figure 2.21). In practice, it has been the lucky combination of elements in certain alloys that has produced the best retentive surfaces. To produce these features, for example by the electrolytic method, usually involves an optimum combination of acid type and concentration, interelectrode distance and current density, all of which have to be determined empirically for each alloy (Box B).

In general, most noble metal alloys cannot be usefully etched to produce adequate retentive features. So far, the alloys which have proved to be the most satisfactory are the base metal, nickel–chromium alloys (Box B). Several contain small amounts of beryllium and, when correctly treated, the etched pattern in these show both undercut cavities and bridged areas (Figures 2.20a and 2.21). These are capable of producing strong bonds throughout the whole treated metal surface and right up to the margins of the flange.

However, beryllium is a particularly dangerous metal to work with, and inhalation of dust containing beryllium can lead to berylliosis in which granulomatous lesions develop in the lungs, leading to shortness of breath, emaciation and even

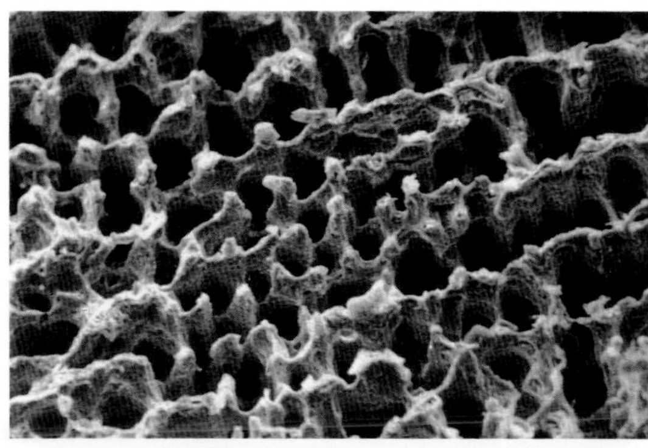

Figure 2.21

SEM of various beryllium-containing, non-precious alloys producing different etch patterns according to composition and dendritic structure. (Magnification ×2030.) (a) Bondiloy (Krupp);

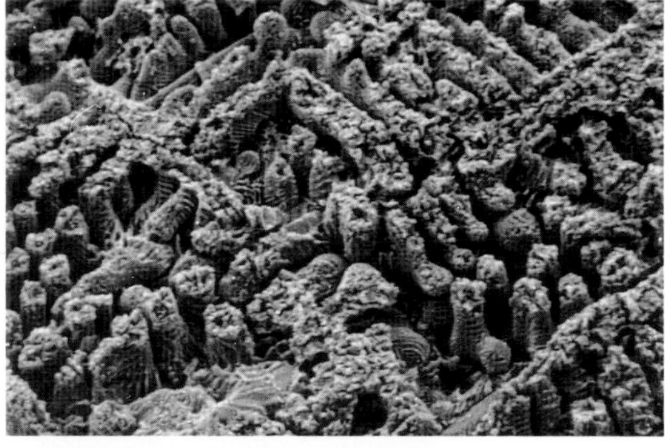

(b) Excelalloy (Exelco);

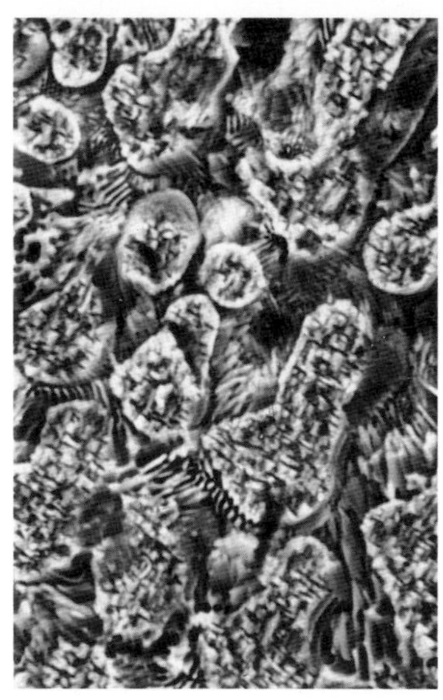

(c) Rexillium III (Jeneric).

BOX B BASE METAL ALLOYS FOR RESIN-BONDED BRIDGES

Nickel–chromium–beryllium alloys

These contain 13–20 per cent chromium, together with small amounts of molybdenum and aluminium. The beryllium content is between 2 and 5 per cent, and there are usually traces of cobalt, copper and titanium.

Common brands

Bak-On NP; Litecast B; Rexillium III; Unitbond.

Treatment to produce retention

After sandblasting with 50 μm alumina followed by ultrasonic cleaning in dilute NH_4OH solution, the alloys are electrolytically etched in 10% H_2SO_4, with or without the presence of methanol, at a current density of between 200 and 300 mA/cm^2 for between 3 and 6 minutes. Ultrasonic cleaning in 18% HCl then follows.

Typical bond strengths

With dimethacrylate cements: 20–30 MPa.

Nickel–chromium alloys

These contain 15–20 per cent chromium, together with small amounts of aluminium, iron, manganese and molybdenum. Some contain boron, niobium, tin and titanium.

Common brands

Biobond C&B; Micro-bond NP2; NCM Alpha; Unibond.

Treatment to produce retention

After sandblasting with 50 μm alumina followed by ultrasonic cleaning in dilute NH_4OH solution, the alloys are electrolytically etched in 0.1–0.5M HNO_3, with or without 2% glacial acetic acid, at a current density of between 250 and 400 mA/cm^2 for 5 minutes. Ultrasonic cleaning in 18% HCl then follows.

Typical bond strengths

With dimethacrylate cements: 20–30 MPa.

Cobalt–chromium alloys

These contain between 30 and 35 per cent chromium, together with small amounts of molybdenum and traces of carbon, iron, manganese, silicon and tungsten. Some contain nickel and titanium.

Commond brands

Bio-Cast; Bondi-loy; Ivotek U; Novarex; Vitallium.

Treatment to produce retention

After sandblasting with 50 μm alumina followed by ultrasonic cleaning, the alloys are electrolytically etched in a mixture of HCl and HNO_3 in methanol at a current density of between 200 and 300 mA/cm^2 for between 7 and 8 minutes. Ultrasonic cleaning in 18% HCl follows, and they are then washed in ethanol and air-dried.

Typical bond strengths

With dimethacrylate cement: 17–20 MPa.

Silver–palladium alloys

These contain 25 per cent palladium together with small amounts of zinc.

Common brands

Albacast; Baker C/B; No. 25; W.L.W.

Treatment to produce retention

After sandblasting with 50 μm alumina followed by ultrasonic cleaning in ethanol, the alloys are electrolytically etched in a solution containing HNO_3, $NaNO_3$ and NaF at a current density of 300 mA/cm^2 for between 1½ and 3 minutes with the etchant ultrasonically stirred. After a water rinse, ultrasonic cleaning in a dilute mixture of H_2SO_4 and H_3PO_4 then follows.

Typical bond strengths

With dimethacrylate cement: 8–15 MPa.

death. Whilst the amounts in these base metal alloys are small and modern air extraction sytems in well-equipped laboratories can take care of the dust and detritus produced by grinding of these alloys, there is a move away from them, using, as an alternative, the beryllium-free nickel–chromium alloys.

Electrolytic etching techniques

There are two methods of electrolytically etching metals and these vary according to whether the etching and cleaning processes take place separately (McLaughlin, 1986), ie the two-step method (Figure 2.22a), or simultaneously, ie the one-step method (Figure 2.22b). For example, the two-step etching programme for Rexillium III—a nickel–chromium–beryllium alloy—using stainless steel electrodes is given as 0.3 A for 3 min in 10% sulphuric acid solution per cm^2 surface to be etched, followed by immersion in 18% hydrochloric acid in an ultrasonic cleaner for 10 minutes. For the one-step method, the same alloy is etched at a rate of 0.45 A for 99 s/cm^2 surface in a premixed solution of sulphuric and hydrochloric acids. Surfaces greater or less than 1 cm^2 require modification of their etching rates using a simple mathematical formula.

The surfaces which are not going to be etched are covered with a hard, brittle, sticky wax and the exposed surfaces are cleaned by sandblasting with 50 μm aluminium oxide abrasive powder before being attached to the anode (Figure 2.23).

On the whole, electrolytic etching is carried out in commercial laboratories using special equipment (Figure 2.24). Recently, compact chairside etching units have appeared. One commercial unit

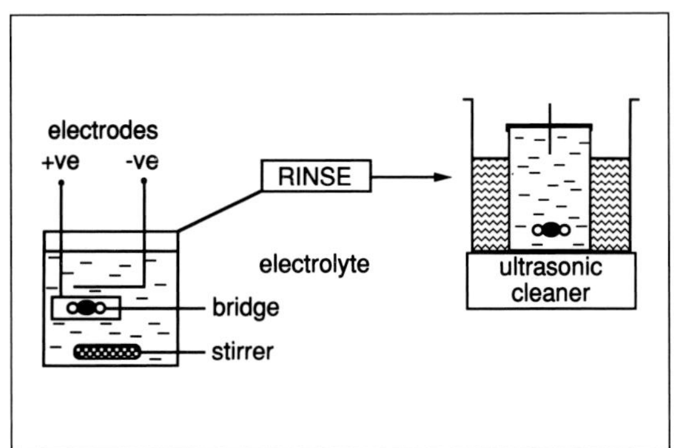

Figure 2.22 a

(a) Diagram of the two-step method for electrolytic etching and cleaning of metals. The electrolyte solution is determined by the alloy being etched (see Box B)—in this instance, for Rexillium III it is 10% sulphuric acid—and is agitated with a magnetic stirrer. The cleaning solution is 18% hydrochloric acid HCl.

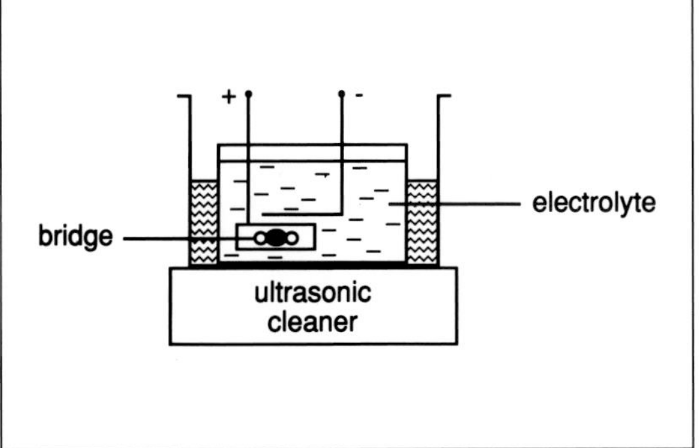

Figure 2.22 b

(b) In the one-step method for Rexillium III, the electrolyte is a premixed solution of sulphuric and hydrochloric acids.

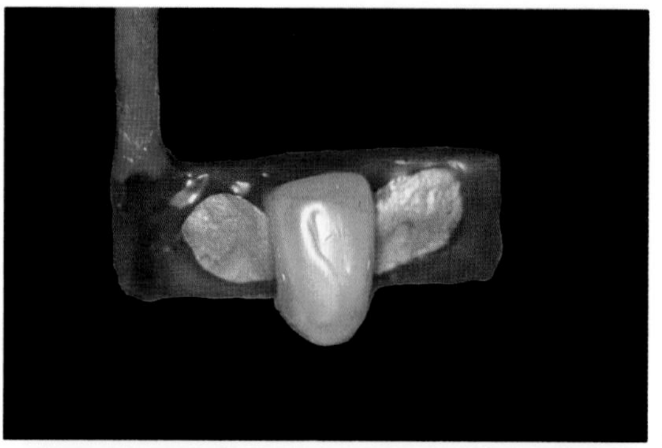

a

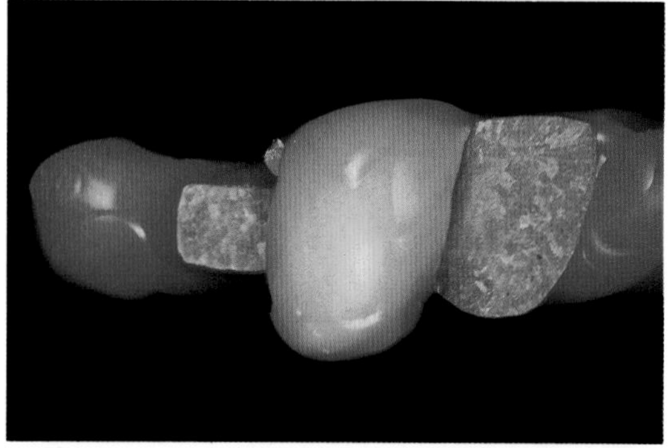

b

Figure 2.23 (a, b)

The surfaces that are not to be etched, such as porcelain pontic facings, are covered with sticky wax. The bridge is attached to the electrode also with sticky wax after the flanges have been cleaned by sandblasting.

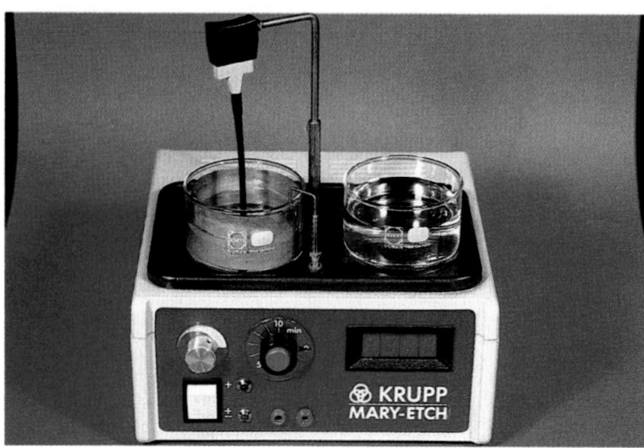

Figure 2.24

An example of a laboratory etching unit—Mary-Etch (Krupp).

(Figure 2.25a) has been tested and shown to produce a satisfactory etch pattern (seen in Figure 2.25c) (Atta et al, 1987a). An etching bath is dispensed with (Figure 2.25b), and the bridge is supported by a metal clip attached to the anode, whereas the cathode comprises a fibre tip soaked in the electrolyte—a weak solution of the acid which will etch the particular alloy. The surface to be etched is flooded with the electrolyte, just touched with the fibre tip and the current is turned on. Depending on the surface area of the bridge to be etched, the procedure should take no more than 10–15 min. This process generates a fair amount of undesirable oxide which could impede bonding to the resin, but the oxide layer can be easily removed by reversing the current.

It is also possible to etch metal without the use of costly electrical equipment, and commercial kits are available to enable this procedure to be carried out in the dental surgery. The acids in these kits are dispensed either in solution, eg Assure-Etch (Williams Gold Refining Co., Inc.) or as a gel, eg Met-Etch (Austenal Dental Products Ltd). They need to be heated to enhance their effectiveness, and great care must be taken in handling these caustic substances—for example, Met-Etch contains 7% hydrofluoric acid. The procedure is summarized in Box C, and a typical etch pattern produced by this method is seen in Figure 2.26e.

Bond-strength values from chemical etching were as good as, if not better than those in the electrolytically etched specimens (Livaditis, 1986; Atta et al, 1987b). Furthermore, chemical etching obviates the need to calculate the surface area of the metal flanges in order to determine the optimum current density required in electrolytic etching. This eliminates one source of error often associated with the latter technique (Hill et al, 1986).

Box C METHOD OF CHEMICALLY ETCHING NON-PRECIOUS METAL SURFACES FOR RESIN-BONDED BRIDGES

1 The bridge is heated in a porcelain furnace at 100°C for 1 minute.
2 A drop of the gel is placed on the flange and teased out to the margins with a plastic (polythene) spatula (Figure 2.27a,b) and left for 1½–2 minutes. During this time, the acid may be seen to work by the amount of bubbles formed and by the change in colour of the gel from white to green and then dark green (Figure 2.27b,c).
3 After this period is up, the gel is rinsed off with tap water and blown dry.
4 Steps 1–3 are repeated four times.
5 Finally, the bridge is cleaned in an ultrasonic bath containing 18% hydrochloric acid solution for 2 minutes and rinsed thoroughly.
6 The bridge should be steam-cleaned to remove all traces of acid before being placed in the mouth.

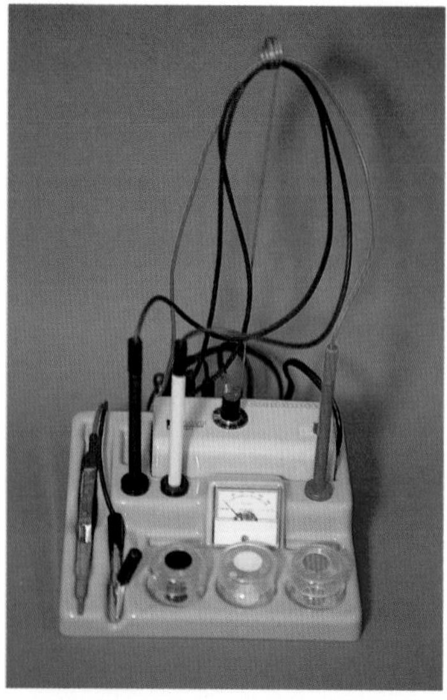

Figure 2.25

(a) An example of a chairside etching unit—Combinette (Wieland).

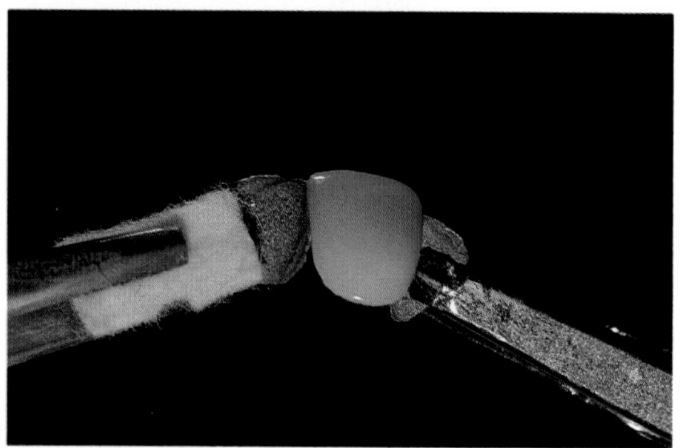

(b) The bridge is clipped to the anode of the chairside etching unit and touched with an absorbent felt tip soaked in the etching solution and connected to the cathode.

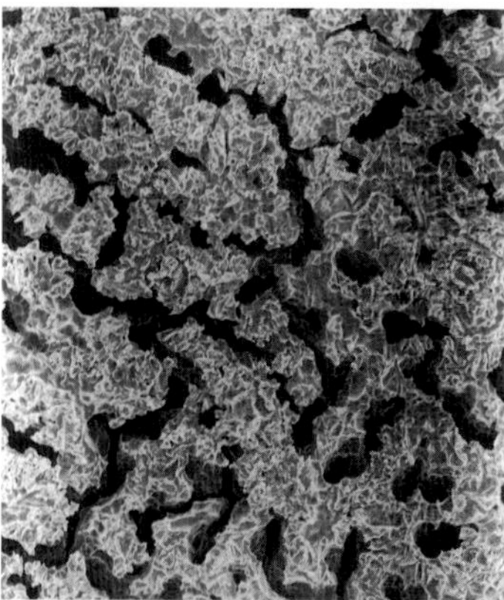

(c) SEM of surface produced by a chairside etching unit. (Magnification ×819.) (Courtesy of Dr O. Atta.)

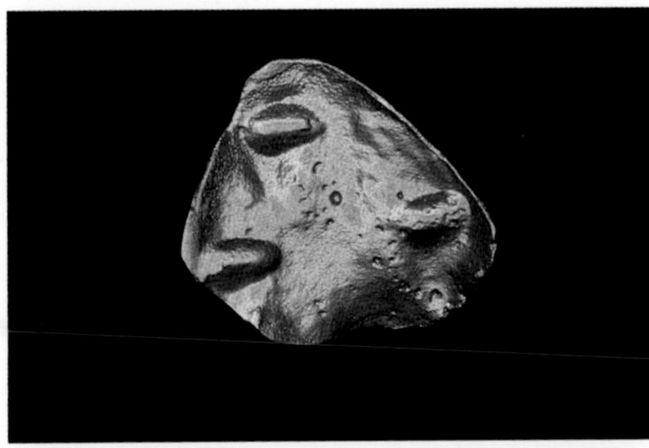

Figure 2.26

(a) Sandblasted and clean surface of metal flange before chemical etching.

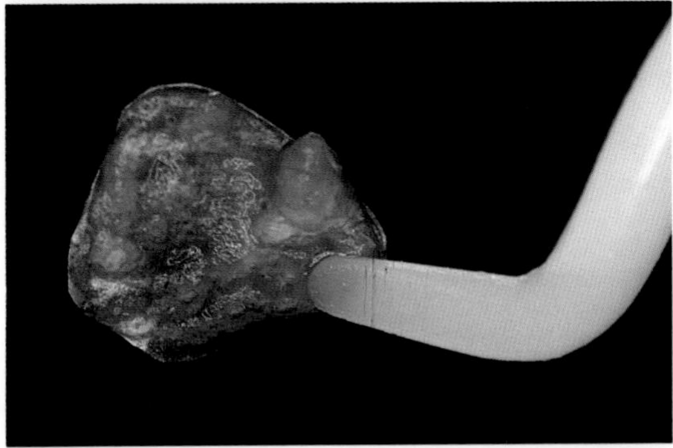

(b) Applying the etching gel (Met-Etch, Austenal) with a plastic instrument. Note the colour change occurring.

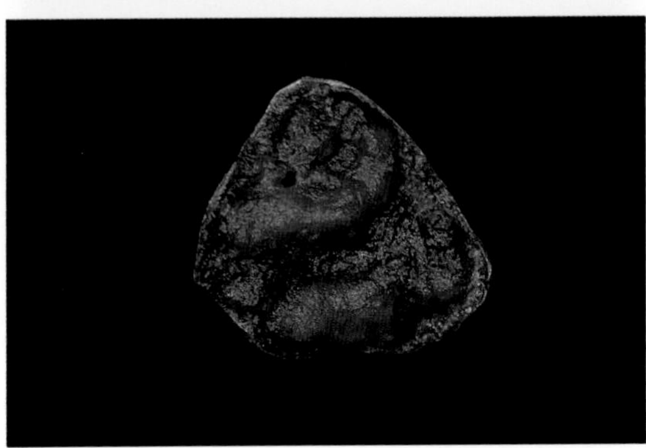

(c) Completion of etch is indicated when the colour of the etching gel turns dark green.

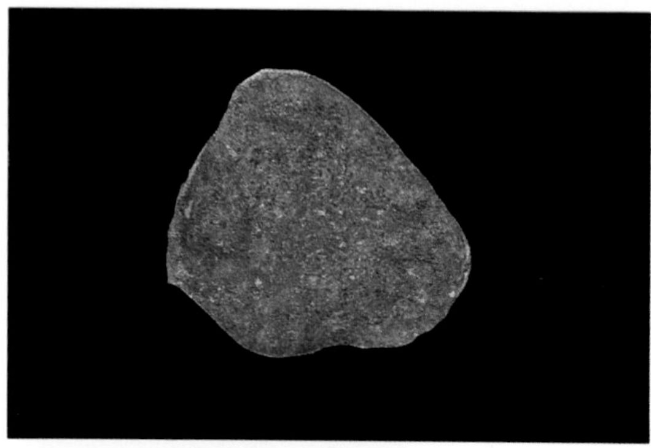

(d) Appearance of etched surface.

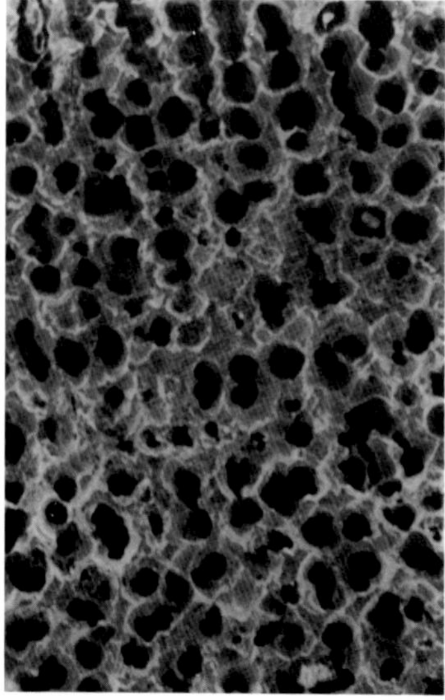

(e) SEM of a chemically etched surface. (Magnification ×819.) (Courtesy of Dr O. Atta.)

Limitations of the etched metal (micromechanical) surface

It is estimated that the total surface available for bonding in electrolytic etching is only 45 per cent, even where undercuts have been created. However, when the resin penetrates into these retentive features and sets, the resistance to tensile dislodging forces is high. The comparative bond strengths between etched and cast-in retention using a common resin is demonstrated in Figure 2.27.

Despite the success of the etched metal design, several reports of difficulties in consistently obtaining good etch patterns, which result in high clinical failure rates, have been received. The high cost of commercial equipment and the vagaries of the technique have delayed universal acceptance of the method.

After the etching process, whether electrolytic or with acid gels, the etched surface is usually examined under a stereomicroscope at magnifications of approximately 50–100 to detect the presence of a definite pattern (Figure 2.28). However,

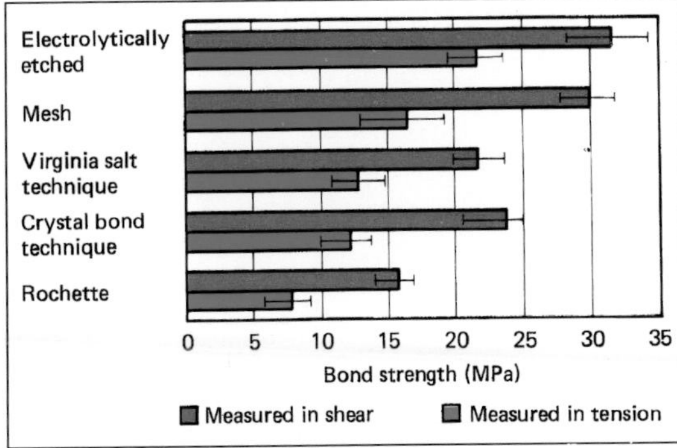

Figure 2.27

Bar graph showing the relative bond strengths tested in shear and in tension of Comspan (Caulk/Dentsply) resin bonded to a nickel–chromium alloy with surface features produced by various techniques.

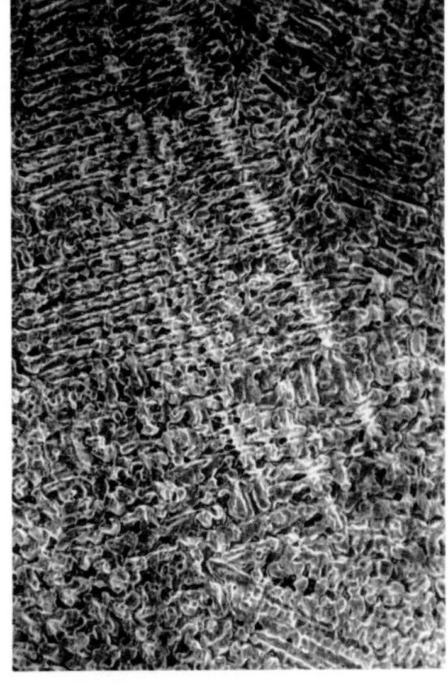

Figure 2.28

SEM of etch pattern at low magnification (×157.5). (Courtesy of Dr O. Atta.)

there are limitations to this approach. It is generally assumed that, if a cross-hatched pattern is seen, then the specimen has been etched satisfactorily, but this can be misleading. For example, Figure 2.29a shows a surface that was judged at low power to have a satisfactory pattern, but at higher magnification the topography appeared to be non-retentive (Figure 2.29b)—probably caused by overetching. Other problems may arise, e.g. at certain current densities electropolishing may occur. Uneven etching, where some sectors of the metal may be inadequately treated, may pass undetected (Figure 2.30). Therefore, the procedure is 'technique sensitive' and dependent on good laboratory practice. One survey in Winnipeg, Canada, showed that the results produced by five participating laboratories indicated a great deal of variation in the quality and consistency of etching (Lyttle et al, 1986). Unfortunately, the survey found that the majority of specimens were unacceptable in terms of display of a good etch pattern, as defined by the investigators, and this suggested poor quality control in the production.

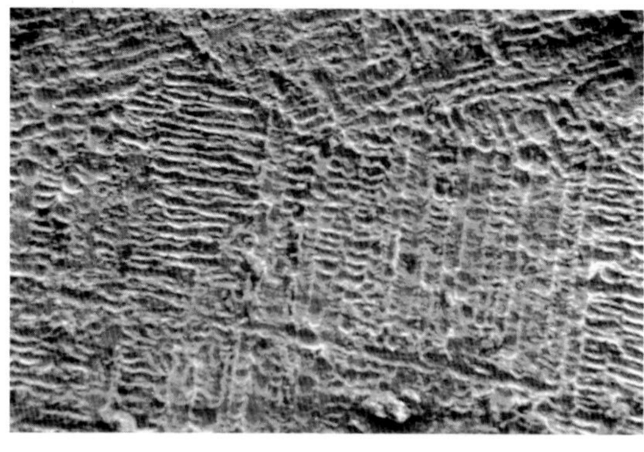

Figure 2.29

(a) Low-power view (×208) of overetched surface which may confuse the inexperienced technician.

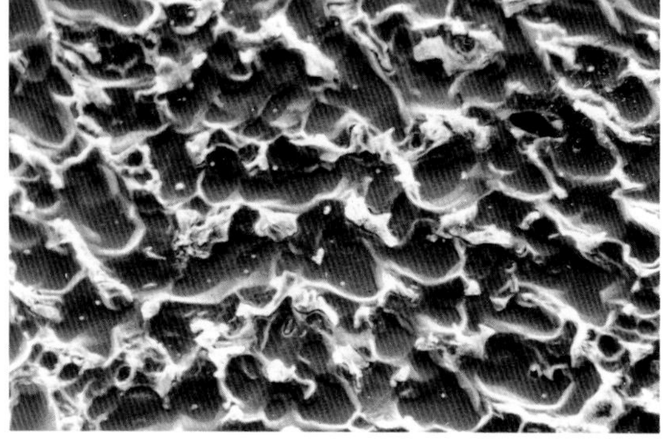

(b) High-power view (×2030) of the same.

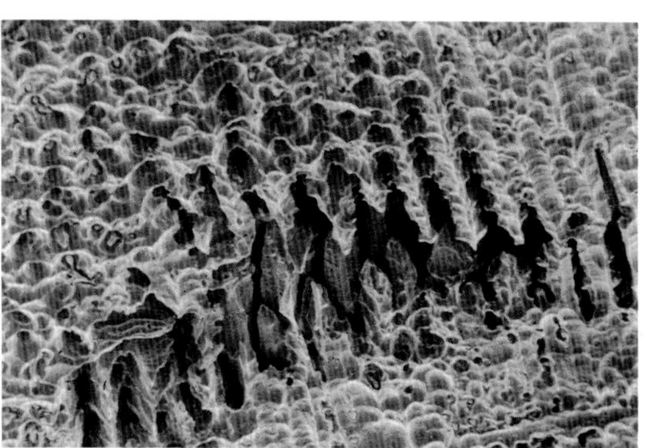

a

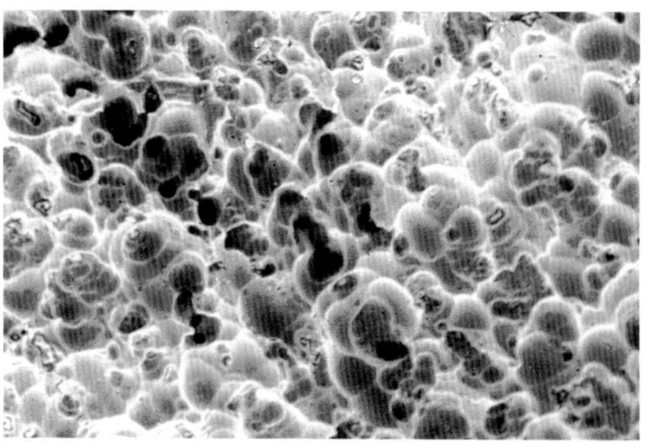

b

Figure 2.30 (a, b)

SEM of unevenly etched surfaces.

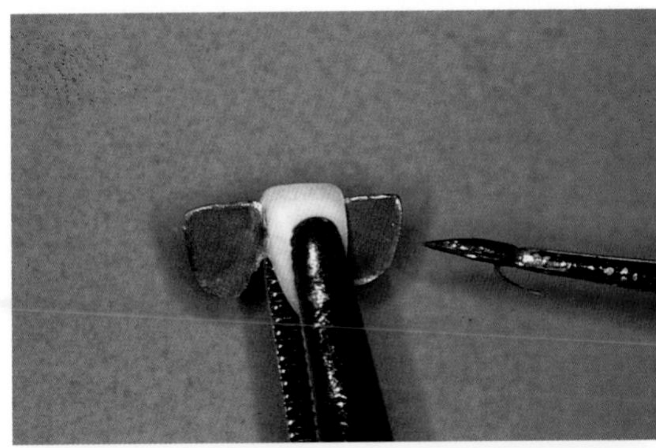

Figure 2.31

(a) Application of Inzoma (Ivoclar) metallic paint.

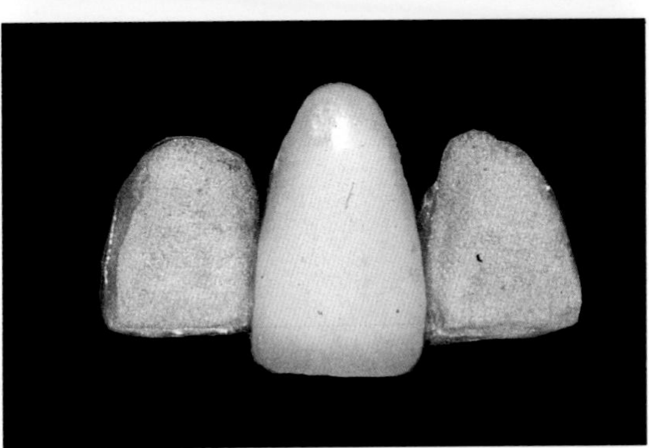

(b) Appearance of treated Inzoma-treated surfaces after baking in a porcelain furnace. (Courtesy of Dr A.N. Stokes.)

Porous metal coatings

Another interesting method of producing a 'pit-and-bead' type of mechanical retention, but at a 'microscopic' level, was reported by Stokes and Tidmarsh (1986, 1987). They used a thin coat of a special metallic 'paint' called Inzoma interzonal material (Ivoclar AG) which produces a porous layer on metal surfaces when treated in a certain manner. Two forms are available, namely Inzoma NP, which is used on non-precious metal alloys, and Inzoma P990 for precious alloys. The material is painted thinly onto the sandblasted metal surface and then fired from room temperature to 970°C with 1½ minutes holding time in an automatic porcelain furnace (Figure 2.31). This produces a porous layer about 20–30 μm thick. As a result of this, the fit surface of the flange to the periphery should be relieved with two layers of die spacer paint. The interzonal material may also be painted on after try-in and adjustment, and before the biscuit stage of porcelain manufacture. The microretentive surface so formed on the metal surface is seen in Figure 2.32.

Sandblasting

The availability of so-called dual affinity or bifunctional resins, ie resins that will chemically bond both to metal and tooth tissue, is the cause of much excitement in the resin-bonding field. With such resins, it is apparently only necessary to sandblast the metal surface, usually with 50–250 μm aluminium oxide abrasive powder, before applying the resin. High bond strengths have been reported, particularly if 250 μm aluminium oxide abrasive is used (Wiltshire 1986a; Atta et al, 1990).

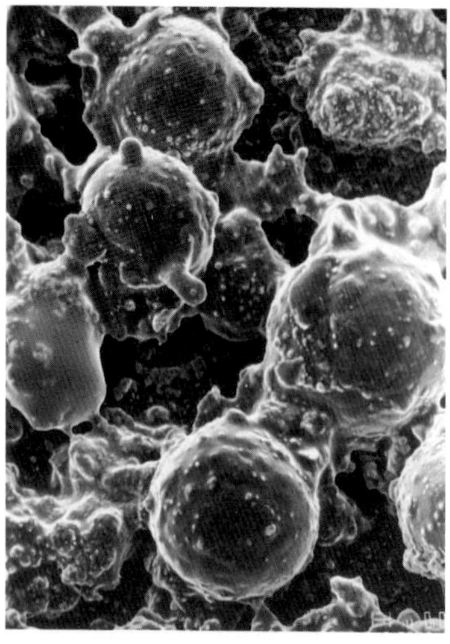

Figure 2.32

(a) SEM of Inzoma NP layer on Rexillium III alloy. (Magnification ×406.)

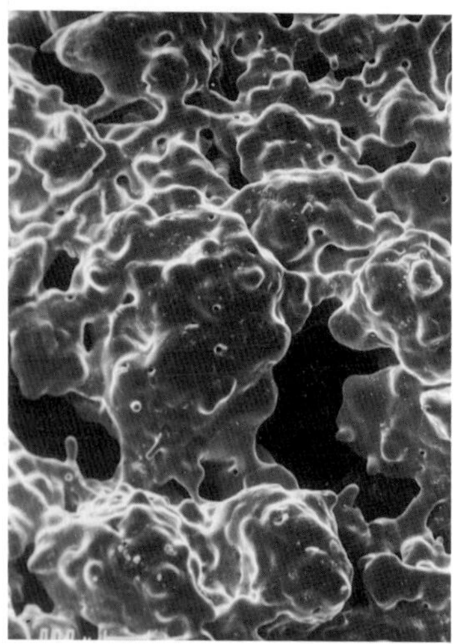

(b) SEM of Inzoma P990 layer on precious alloy (×406).

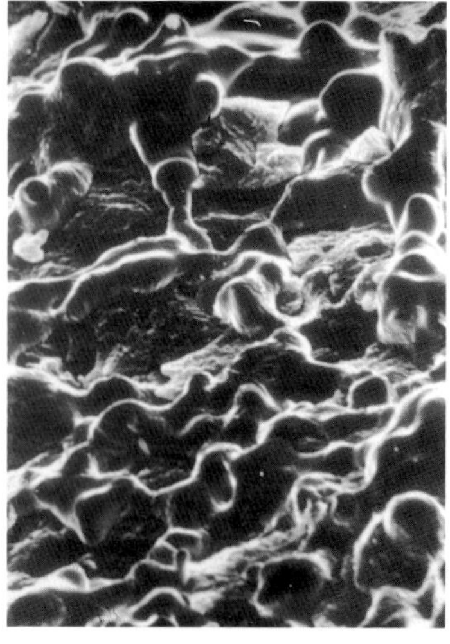

(c) The same with resin trapped within the pores. (Courtesy of Dr A.N. Stokes.)

The abrasive powder is fed through an air brush (Figure 2.33) operating at pressures of 3–35 kg/cm^2 which produces minute irregularities on metal surfaces; this effectively increases the surface area and provides irregularities for micromechanical bonding (Figure 2.34b). The technique is particularly applicable to nickel–chromium alloys. The nozzle tip should be held about 5 mm from the flange and played across the surface until a matt finish appears (Figure 2.34a). This is then followed by ultrasonic cleaning for 60 seconds.

A particular bonding resin (Figure 2.35), Panavia EX (Kuraray), is reputed to show a strong bond to a sandblasted metal surface, but it is claimed that even better results can be achieved if the metal has an oxide film on its surface (Atta et al, 1990). This can be carried out simply by immersing the metal in an aqueous solution of 3% sulphuric acid and 1% potassium permanganate for 15 seconds.

An instrument called the EZ Oxisor (Towa Co.), which is a simple hand-held battery-operated oxidation device, may be used (Figure 2.36a). The brush is dipped in an oxidizing agent and, when the current is turned on, nascent oxygen is produced which then reacts with the metal surface to produce a film of oxide (Figure 2.36b). This oxide film is supposed to improve wetting between Panavia EX and the metal and consequently to enhance the bond.

Surfaces capable of promoting chemical bonding

With all the foregoing methods, retention of the composite resin to the metal is solely mechanical and therefore susceptible to stress fatigue. It would be highly desirable to achieve true chemical bonding of resin to metal and two methods of pretreating the metal surface to encourage chemical 'attractiveness' to bonding resins have been tried.

Tin-plated flange

Successful bonding of composite resin to tin-plated metal flanges is possible. The pioneers of this technique for resin-bonded bridges are H. van der Veen and his co-workers at the University of Groningen (Veen et al, 1986, 1988a,b) who achieved higher bond strengths of resin to tin-plated metal than resin to electrolytically etched metal. The coating of tin is deposited on the metal by electrochemical means (Figure 2.37a). Owing to the crystalline texture of the layer, an increased surface area for micromechanical retention is possible (Figure 2.37b,c). The tin surface is sometimes oxidized to enhance chemical bonding with the composite resin.

Tin plating is most suited to gold or gold–silver–palladium alloys, and not so effective with non-precious alloys. Commercial units are available which simplify the process, eg Micro Tin which is a hand-held battery-operated, compact unit (Figure 2.38), and the OVS and Kura Ace systems (Figures 2.39 and 2.40) which are used at the chairside or in the laboratory. As with the electrolytic etching technique, careful control of voltage, current density and rate of plating is essential to produce a good surface. Sandblasting of the surface with 50 µm aluminium oxide before plating is advisable. The tin surface oxidizes readily either by heating in air in a furnace or by using the EZ Oxisor and, again, this is said to improve bonding.

Silicon oxide coatings

Another method of producing a chemical linkage between resin and metal is through the intermediary of a layer of silicon oxide—the so-called 'SiO_x-C' layer (Musil and Tiller, 1984). The Silicoater technique, as it is known, involves the vaporization of a silane (tetraethoxysilane) in a propane–air flame. The molecules of decomposed silane are then 'welded' in very thin layers onto the sandblasted metal surface (Figure 2.41), although essentially the retention is believed to be mechanical in nature, by virtue of the irregularities of the sandblasted surface (Hero et al, 1987). A grain size for the sand of 250 µm was found to produce the best surface for strong bonding to the 'silicoat' layer (Peutzfeldt and Asmussen, 1988).

The thickness of the SiO_x-C layer is approximately 100–1000 nm (Figure 2.42). The essential nature of this layer is glassy, but the presence of carbon and hydroxyl groups reduces the number of silicon bonds rendering the layer less rigid and more elastic. This elasticity helps to distribute strains, from temperature variations and shearing forces in the mouth, over an extensive area thus preserving the bond between resin and metal (Hansson, 1989). After cooling, a film of silane solution is painted on the coated surface and dried before applying the composite resin-luting cement. Because the resin cannot adhere directly to the silicoat layer, the silane film is necessary as a coupling agent. The total thickness of the silicoat and silane film is less than 1 μm and will not obstruct the seating of the casting. The technique is summarized in Box D.

This is perhaps one of the most promising developments in the search for true chemical bonding of resins to metal. The main drawback is that an expensive furnace attached to propane gas cylinders is required for the vaporizing and coating processes. An alternative electric furnace (see Figure 2.41a), the Silicoater MD which dispenses with the gas cylinders, has recently been introduced.

All-porcelain bridge

The solution to the problem of occlusal interferences posed by the lingual placement of cast-metal, resin-bonded bridges has been manifest in the use of porcelain retainers placed labially/buccally or approximally.

Thin veneers of porcelain have become increasingly popular in recent years for improving the appearance of badly discoloured, chipped or malformed teeth. Examples are the Mirage (Chameleon Dental Products Inc.) and Cerinate (Den-Mat Corp.) dental porcelain systems. Minimal tooth preparation is necessary and these veneers, or laminates as they are sometimes called, are placed on the labial surfaces of teeth, thus avoiding any conflict with the opposing occlusal surfaces (Ibsen and Strassler, 1986). A porcelain pontic is fused to the retainer veneers (Figure 2.43a). Retention for the bonding resin is created on the fit surface by acid etching, usually with a strong solution of hydrofluoric acid (Figure 2.43b). The etched surface is then steam-cleaned and primed with a silane coupling agent before the luting resin is applied.

Some examples of all-porcelain veneer bridges are illustrated in Figures 2.44–2.46.

A variant of the all-porcelain bridge is seen in Figure 2.47. Here, the porcelain pontic is retained not by thin veneers, but by porcelain inlays supported within their corresponding approximal inlay preparations.

No published clinical results are available for the all-porcelain resin-bonded bridge, and it is doubtful whether this bridge, especially the veneer type, can sustain the forces in the mouth. Besides the fragility of porcelain, particularly at the junction with the pontic, the other disadvantage is that the embrasures are often obliterated in the interest of strength, and this may often compromise the desire for good aesthetics and the ability to be cleansed. Recently, stronger porcelains, such as the fibre-reinforced types, are being introduced and may well solve the problem of fatigue stress of porcelain.

BOX D SILICON OXIDE TREATMENT

The deposition of silicon oxide is carried out in the Silicoater (Kulzer). The steps are as follows:

1 Sandblast the metal surface with 250 μm grain size carborundum at a blasting pressure of 4 bar. Sandblasting time for precious metal alloys is 10–15 seconds per surface, and for non-precious alloys 30 seconds per surface.
2 Rinse the sandblasted surface in Siliclean (Kulzer).
3 Mount the bridge in the Silicoater (Figure 2.42a) and do a dry run without the flame.
4 Adjust the propane–air mixture until the correct flame is obtained then start the run for 3–5 minutes.
5 After cooling, paint the coated surface with silane solution, Silicoup (Kulzer) followed by air drying for 2–5 minutes.

The treated metal surfaces are now ready to receive the bonding resin and this must be achieved within 24 hours because the silane bond is relatively unstable.

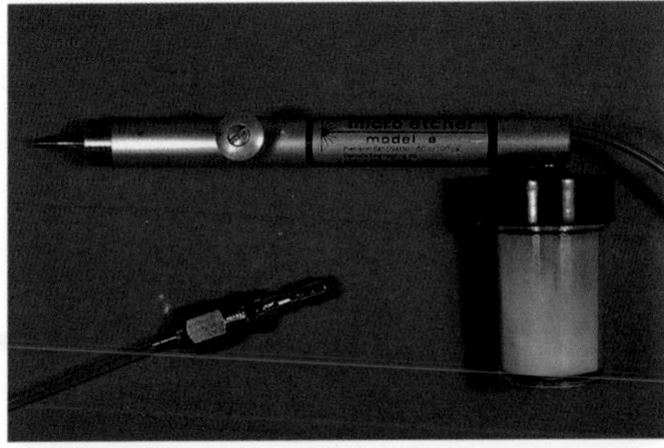

Figure 2.33

Micro Etcher (Danville Engineering) precision sandblasting instrument.

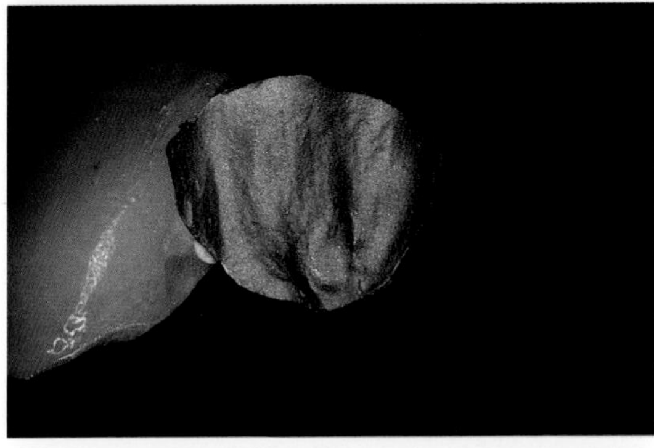

Figure 2.34

(a) Matt surface on metal after sandblasting.

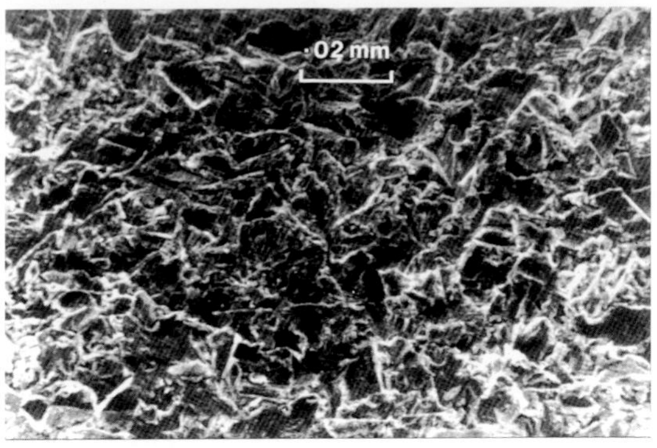

(b) SEM of sandblasted surface (magnification ×2030) .

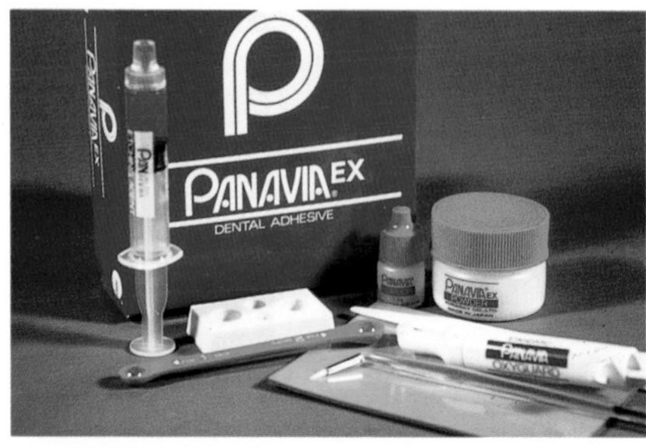

Figure 2.35

Panavia EX (Kuraray)—a popular chemically adhesive cement.

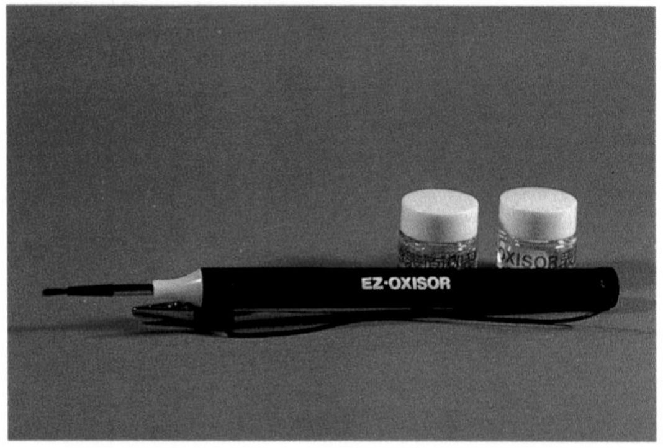

Figure 2.36

(a) EZ Oxisor (Towa Co.)—battery-operated oxidizing pen.

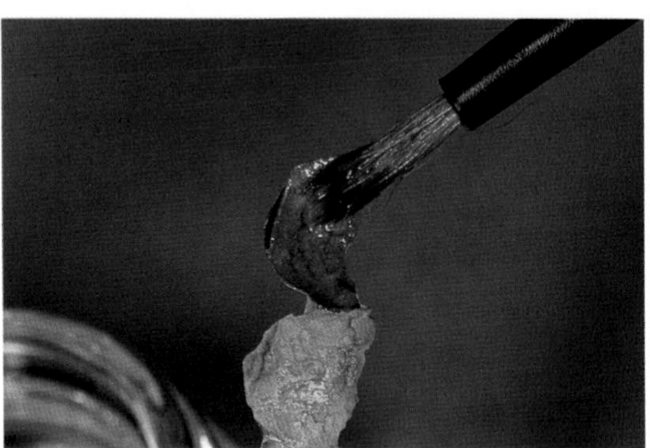

(b) Oxidizing a sandblasted surface with the EZ Oxisor.

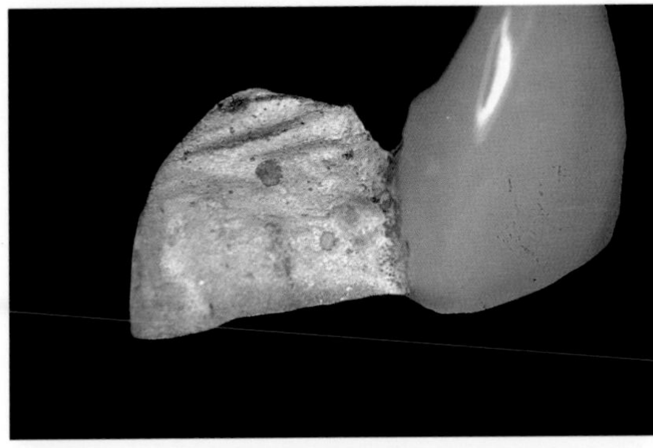

Figure 2.37

(a) Appearance of a tin-plated surface.

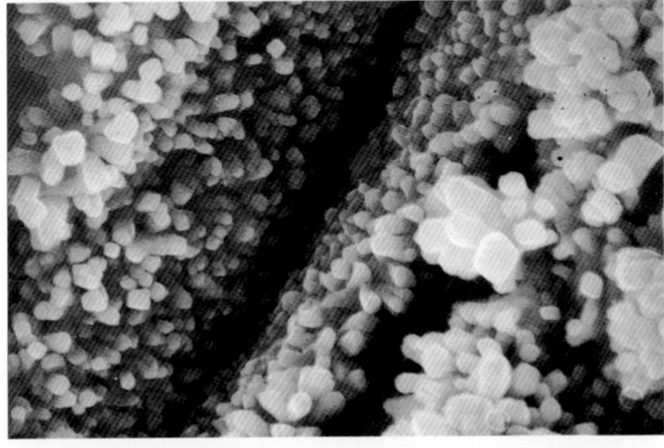

(b) SEM of crystalline tin layer at 12 V plating impedance. (Magnification ×12180.)

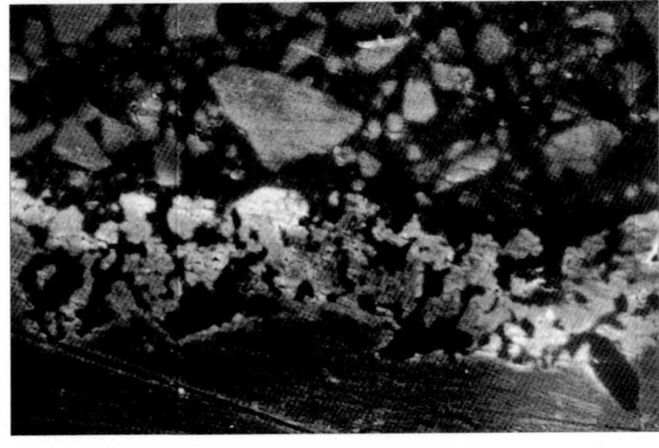

(c) SEM of section through composite resin (top), tin layer (middle) and metal (bottom). Field width is approximately 25 μm. (Courtesy of Dr H. van der Veen.)

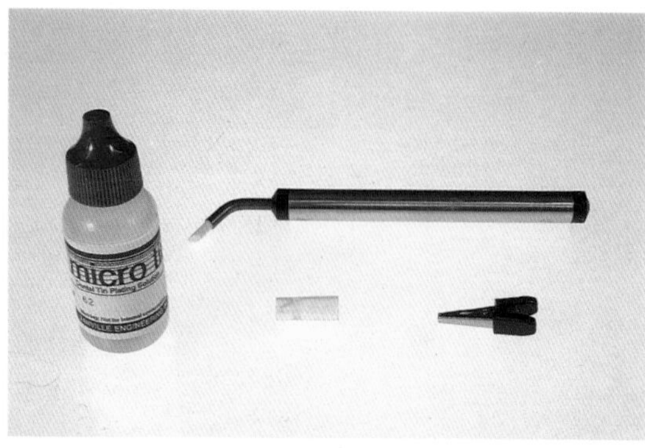

Figure 2.38

(a) Micro Tin (Danville Engineering)—battery-operated precision tin-plating system.

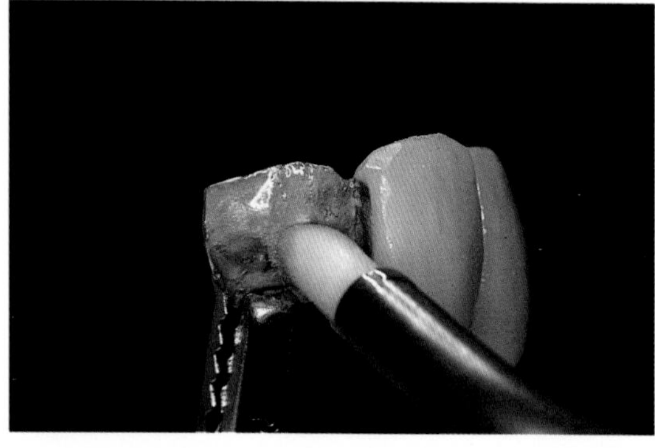

(b) Felt plating tip saturated with tin solution applied to metal surface.

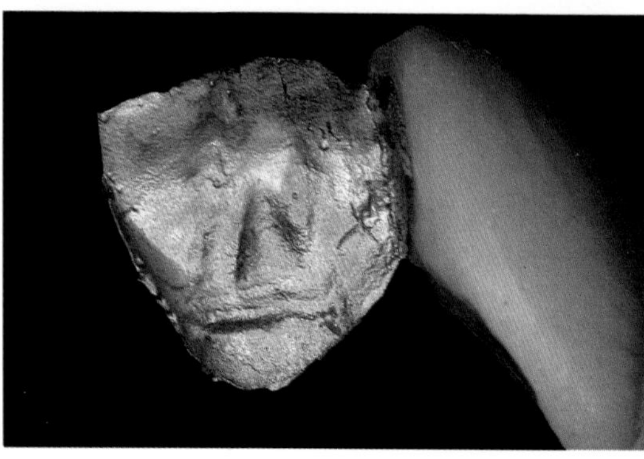

(c) Appearance of tin-plated surface.

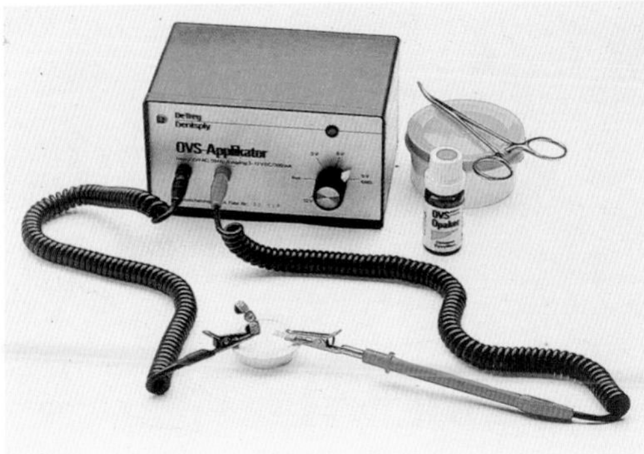

Figure 2.39

The OVS (Dentsply) tin-plating system.

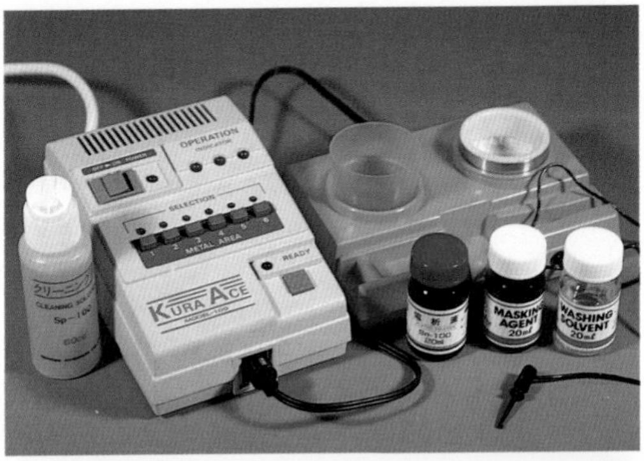

Figure 2.40

(a) Kura Ace (Kuraray) tin-plating system.

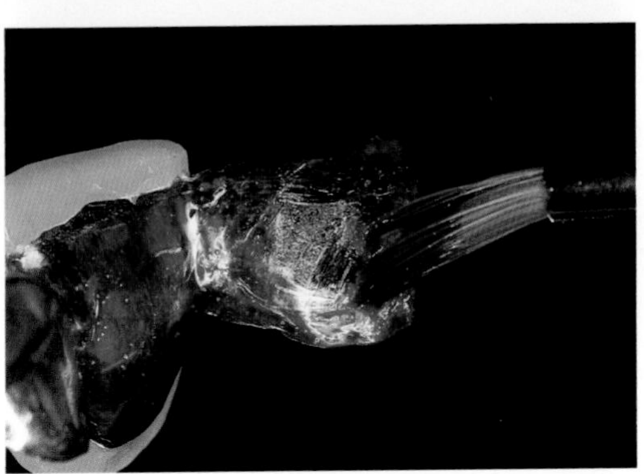

(b) Surfaces that are not to be plated are protected with a layer of varnish.

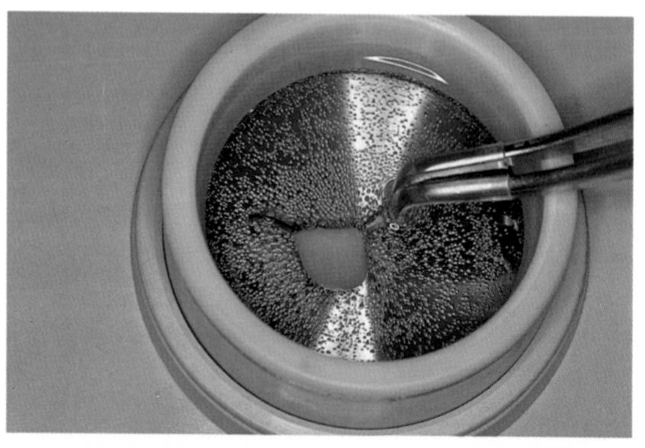

(c) The bridge is held in a pair of locking tweezers connected to the plating unit and immersed in a jar of tin solution. Bubbles indicate plating activity.

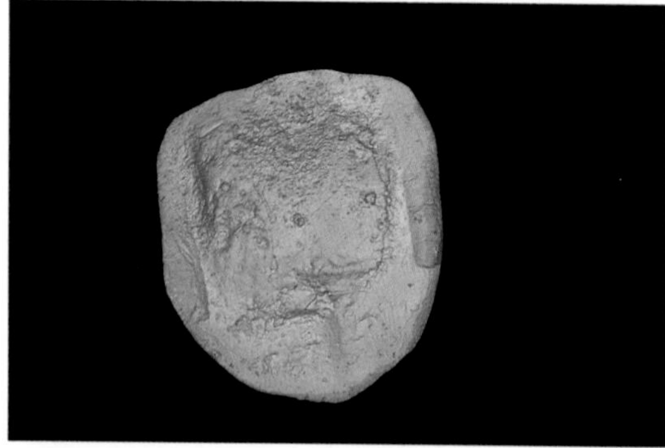

(d) Appearance of tin-plated surface produced by the Kura Ace unit.

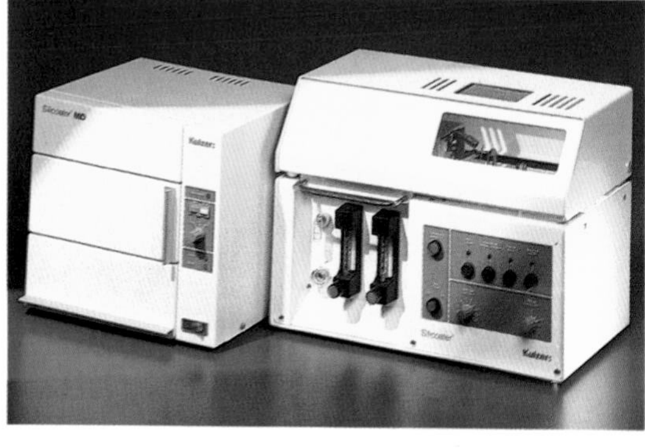

Figure 2.41

(a) Left: the Silicoater MD (Kulzer) electric furnace which dispenses with the propane gas cylinders associated with the older Silicoater unit on the right.

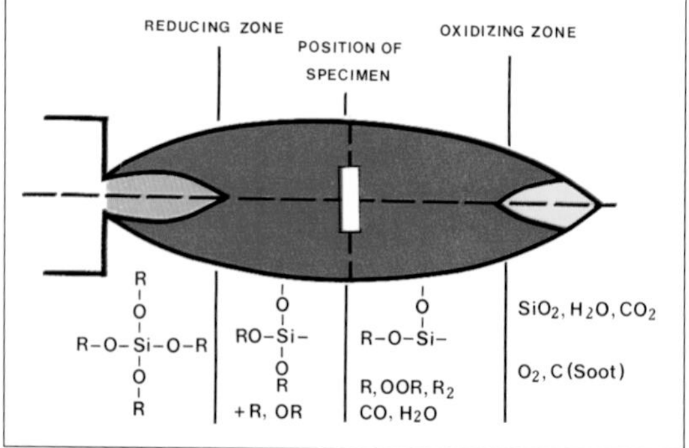

(b) Diagram of the propane gas flame in the Silicoater unit which vaporizes the silane solution and forms the 'silicoat' layer on the metal. (Courtesy of Kulzer & Co. GmbH.)

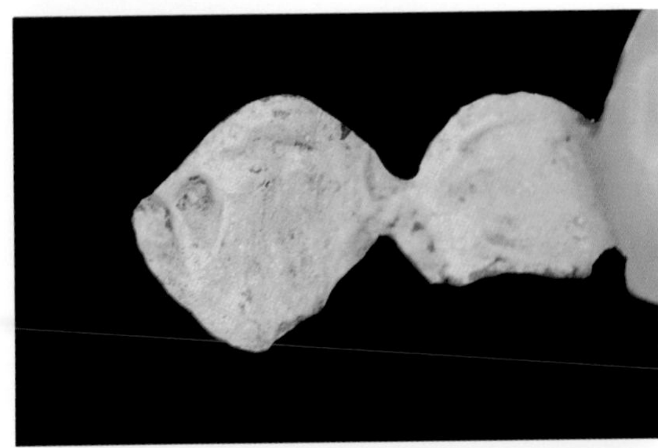

Figure 2.42

(a) Appearance of the 'silicoated' metal flanges.

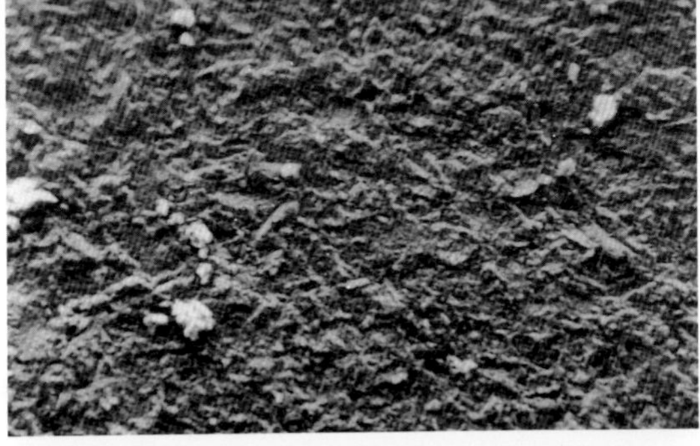

(b) SEM of a 'silicoated' layer. (Magnification ×4060.)

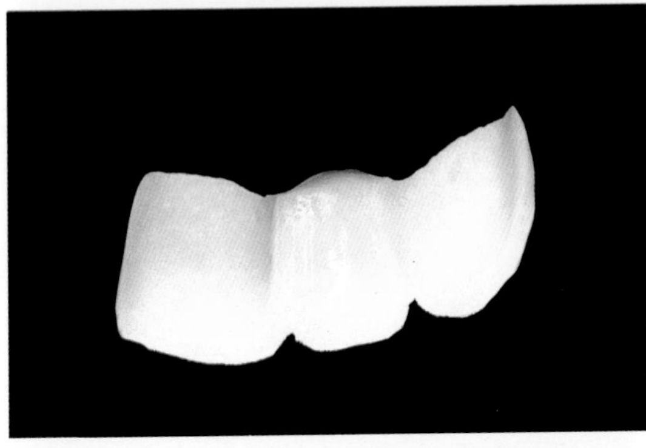

Figure 2.43

(a) All-porcelain bridge using porcelain veneers as retainers.

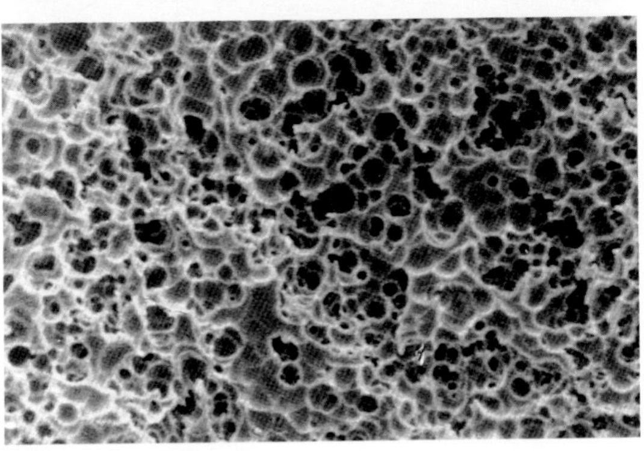

(b) SEM of the etched surface of a porcelain veneer. (Magnification ×4160.)

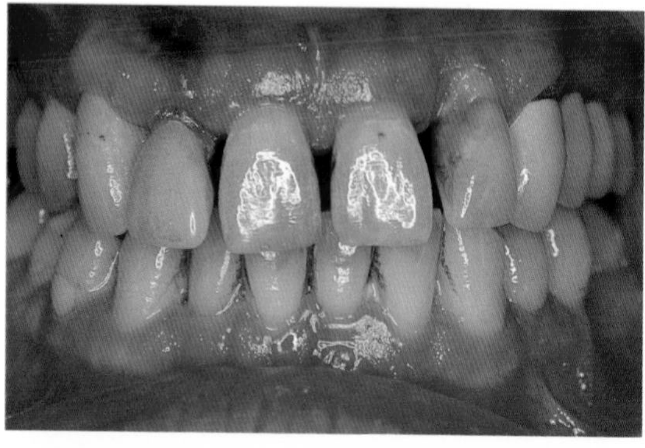

Figure 2.44

(a) The upper left and right lateral incisors of this patient were due to be extracted for periodontal reasons.

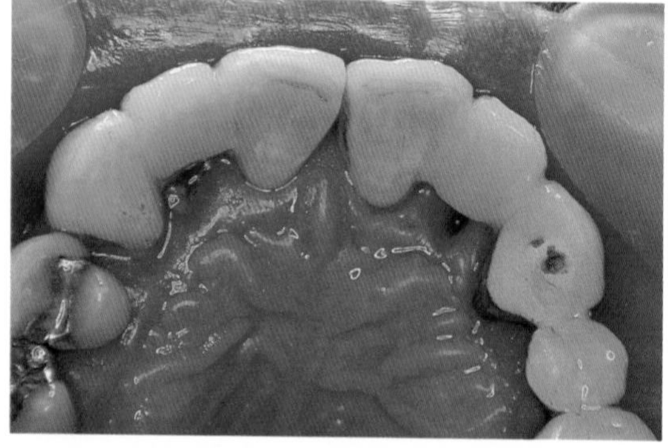

(b) After extraction, two all-porcelain bridges with labially placed porcelain veneer retainers were immediately fitted.

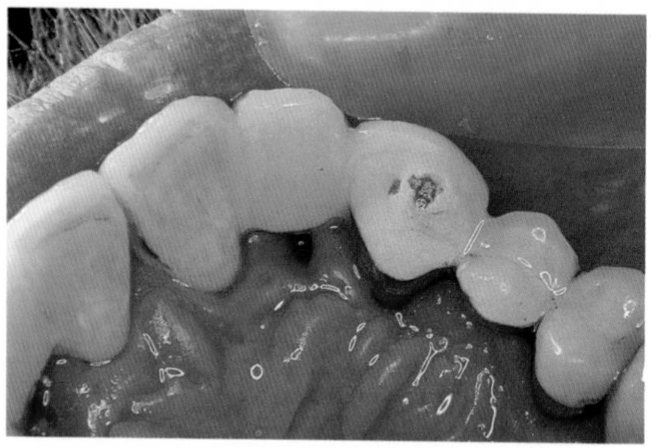

(c) The porcelain retainer bonded well to the etched surface of the existing upper left canine which had a metal–ceramic crown.

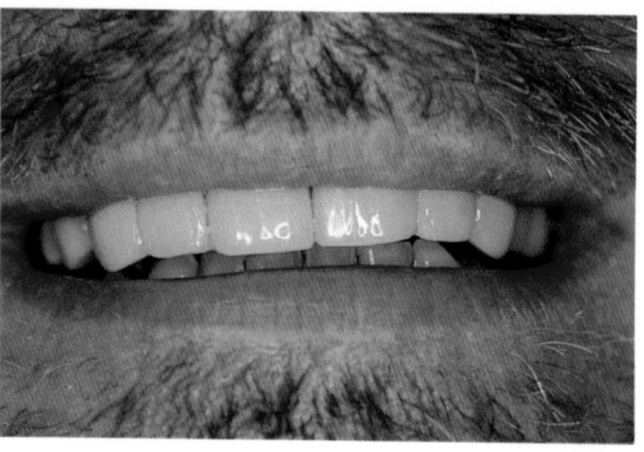

(d) The completed bridges seen through the patient's half-smile. (Courtesy of Dr E. Lynch.)

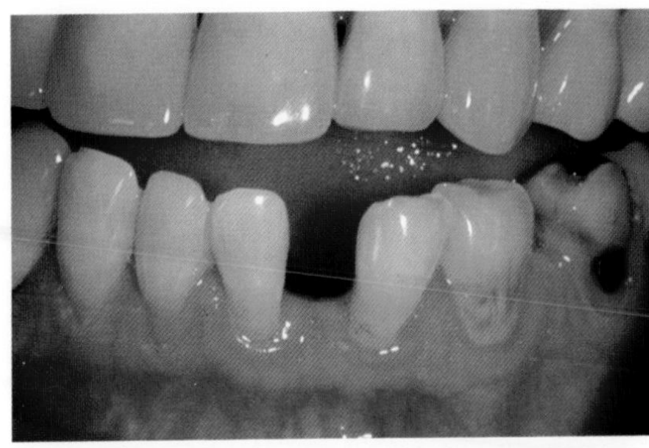

Figure 2.45

Replacement of a lower left central incisor with an all-porcelain bridge. (a) Preoperative appearance;

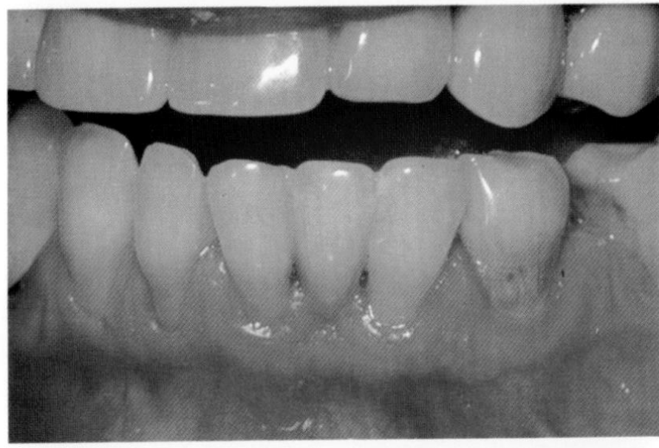

(b) the bridge in place;

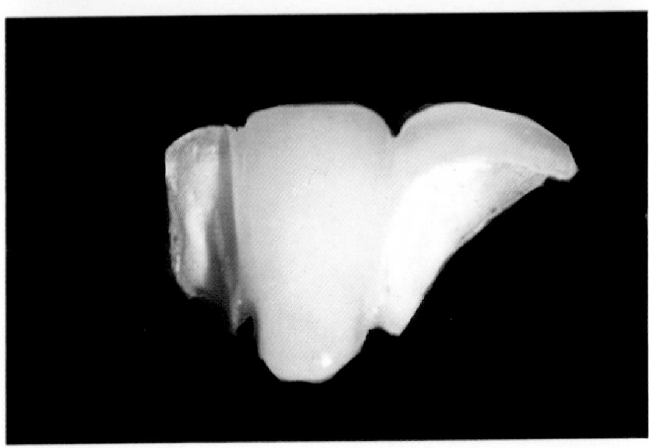

(c) close-up of the bridge showing lingually placed veneer retainers;

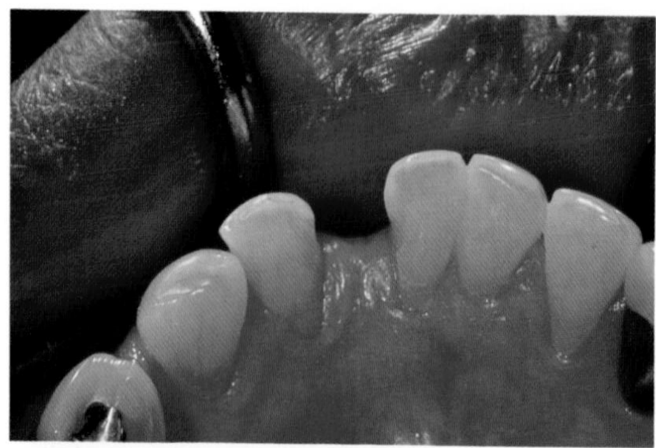

(d) preoperative—lingual view;

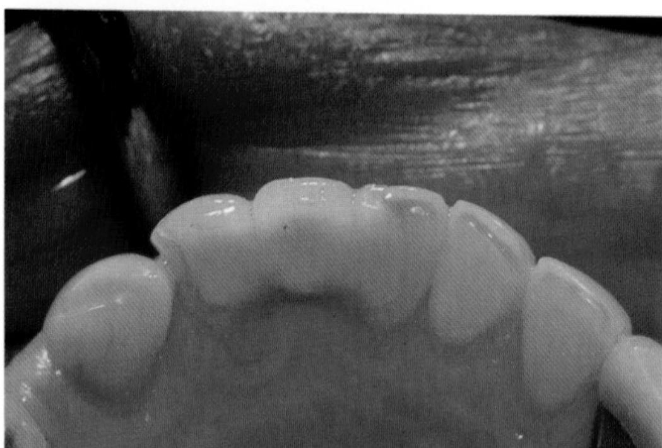

(e) the bridge in place—lingual view. (Courtesy of Dr J.N. Nasedkin.)

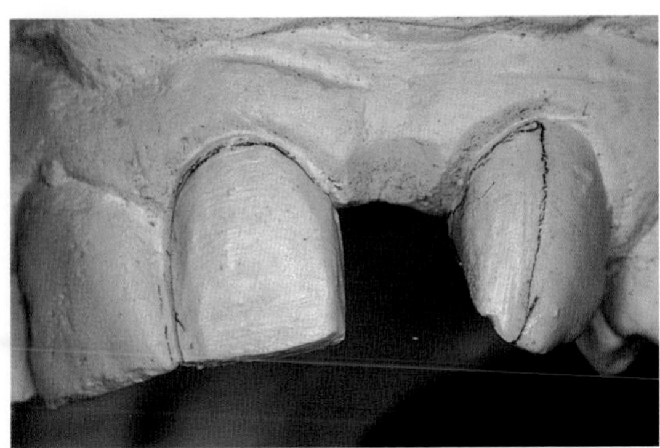

Figure 2.46

(a) Working plaster model for an all-porcelain bridge with labial veneers replacing upper left lateral incisor.

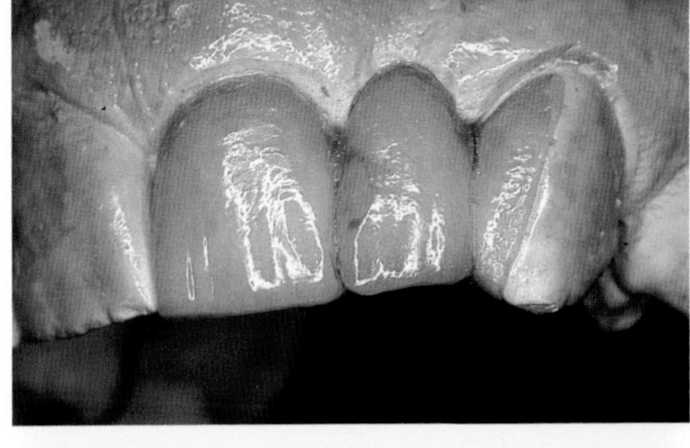

(b) The completed bridge: the left retainer partially covers the canine to avoid wrapping over the labial bulge of the tooth and encroaching on an undercut region.

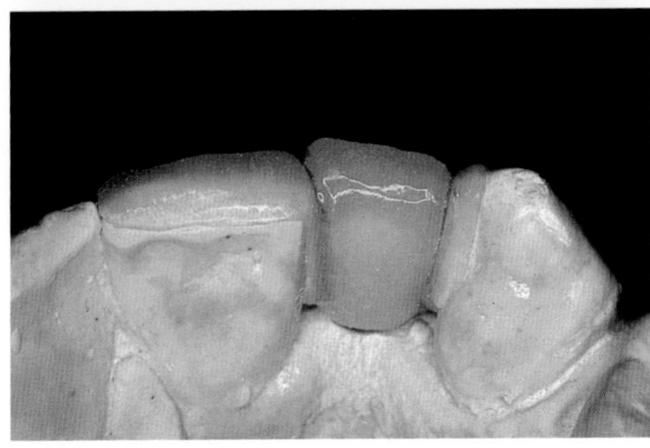

(c) Lingual aspect of the bridge. (Courtesy of Mr M. Gill.)

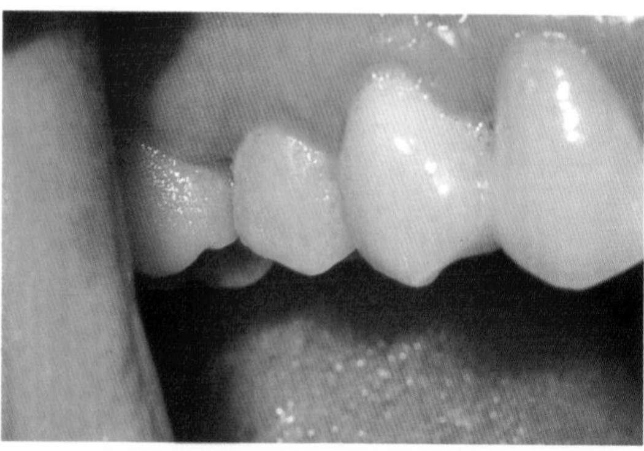

Figure 2.47

(a) All-porcelain bridge replacing upper right first premolar.

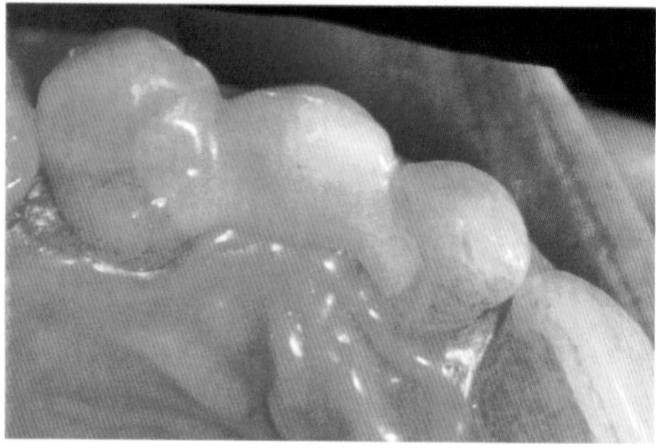

(b) The bridge is retained by etched porcelain inlays. (Courtesy of Dr J.N. Nasedkin.)

3 Bonding to tooth enamel

It seems paradoxical that the simple concept of an adhesive bridge should be fraught with so many difficulties to frustrate the unwary operator. The mouth has often been described as having a destructive nature where dental materials are concerned. In this warm, humid environment, micro-organisms proliferate and their end-products may adversely affect the quality of the resin adhesives or destroy the enamel substrate (adherend) through the process of dental caries. With an average biting force of 56.5 kg (554 N) or 125 pounds, chewing stresses may reach 170 kg/cm^2 (17 MN/m^2) or 2418 lbf/in^2 and over for a single thrust of a molar cusp on something as firm as a carrot. Extreme temperature changes during eating may be transmitted rapidly via the metal flanges of the bridge to put stress on the resin bond. Tooth surfaces are frequently contaminated with bacterial plaque and small amounts of other organic and inorganic material. Water abounds and is the prime destroyer of adhesive bonds. It is quite amazing that any resin-bonded bridge should stay in place!

Etching the enamel surface

No matter how smooth the tooth surface appears to the naked eye, microscopically it invariably appears rough (Figure 3.1a). A degree of retention can occur but mechanical interlocking may be enhanced considerably by etching which creates greater irregularities and, provided the adhesive is able to penetrate completely, very strong bonds may be formed.

The application of a weak inorganic acid to the surface of clean enamel for a short period of time produces changes in the enamel in two distinct ways. Superficially, a layer of enamel about 10 μm deep is removed. This layer may contain plaque, surface and subsurface organic pellicles, and some enamel prisms. Next, selective decalcification up to 120 μm deep may occur, producing pores and crevices within the enamel. Thus acid etching may aid bonding to enamel by:

1 The removal of debris.
2 Raising the free surface energy of the enamel to exceed the surface tension of the bonding resin allowing thorough wetting of the surface.
3 Producing spaces or etch patterns (eg Figure 3.1b) into which the resin may penetrate to form tag-like extensions (Figure 3.1c) and interlock when set.
4 Increasing the surface area of enamel available to the bonding resin.

Types of acids

Phosphoric acid is the most widely used etching solution or etchant in commercial bonding kits and is available either as a liquid or a thixotrophic gel. Research has shown that there is no difference in the etch patterns produced by a liquid or gel etchant (Simonsen and Tierney, 1985); nor was there any significant difference in the depth of penetration of the resin tags or in the shear strength of the enamel–resin bond (Walker and Vann, 1984). The only advantage in using a gel etchant is the greater control available when applying and limiting it to a particular region of the enamel surface and reducing the chances of spillage onto exposed dentine, soft tissues or rubber dam clamps.

The strength of acid in these kits may vary between 30% and 50% by weight and 37% appears to be the most favoured figure among manufacturers. At these concentrations, the acids, when applied to the enamel surface for up to 1 minute,

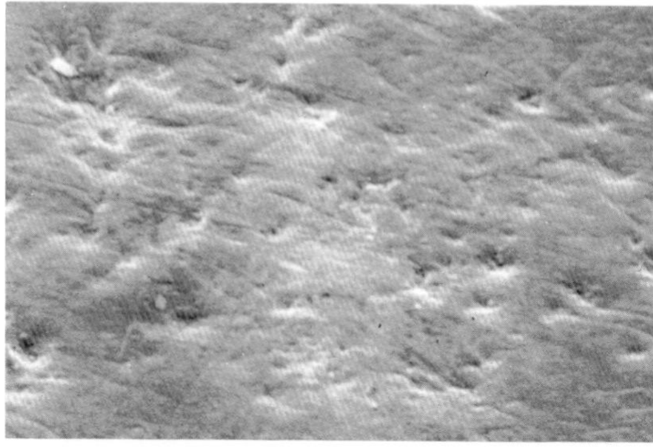

Figure 3.1

(a) SEM of unetched enamel surface.

(b) SEM of type I etch pattern showing 'honeycomb' appearance.

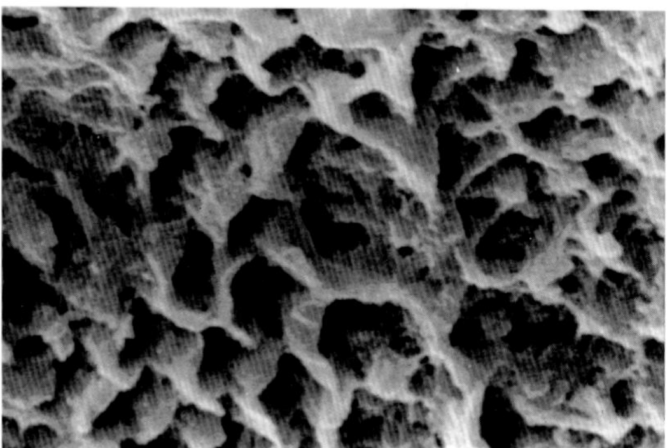

(c) SEM of resin tags (after removal of enamel) formed by the penetration of resin into the 'honeycomb'.

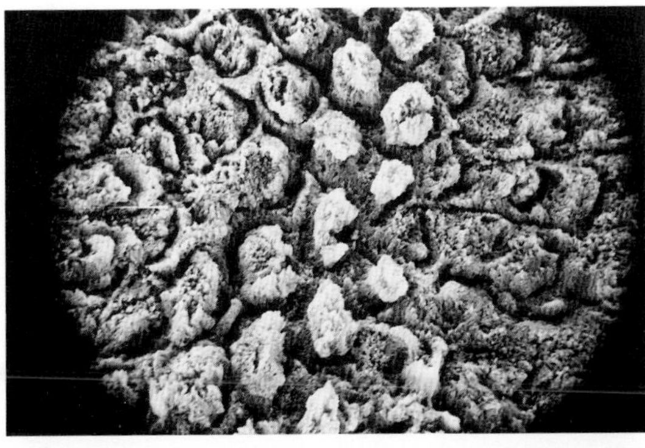

Figure 3.1

(d) Type 2 etch pattern showing preferential removal of enamel prism peripheries. (Magnification ×6090.)

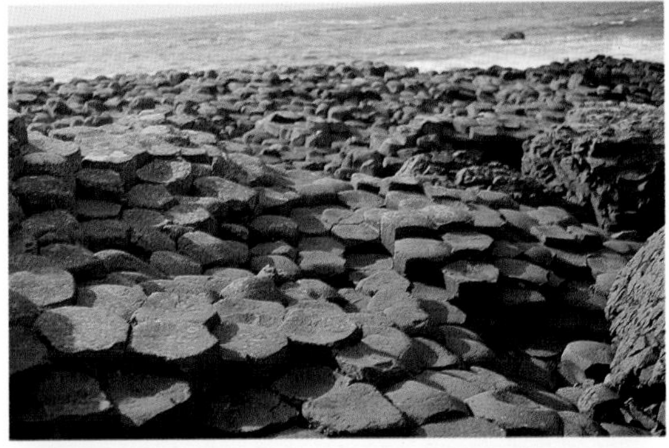

(e) The 'Giant's Causeway' natural basalt formation in County Antrim, Northern Ireland. (Courtesy of Dr M. Levinkind.)

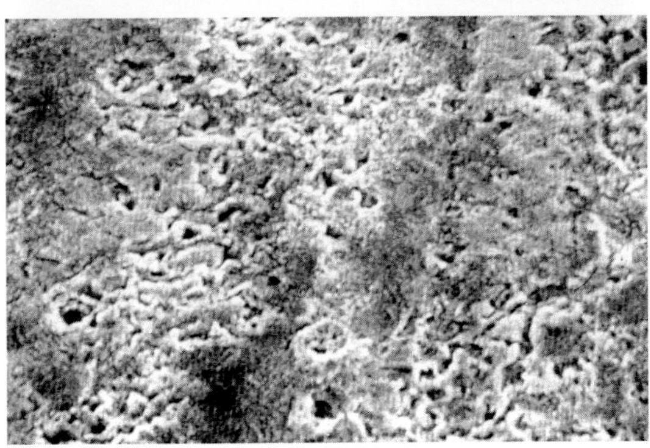

(f) SEM of type 3 etch pattern showing a nondescript appearance. (Magnification of SEMs at ×2030.)

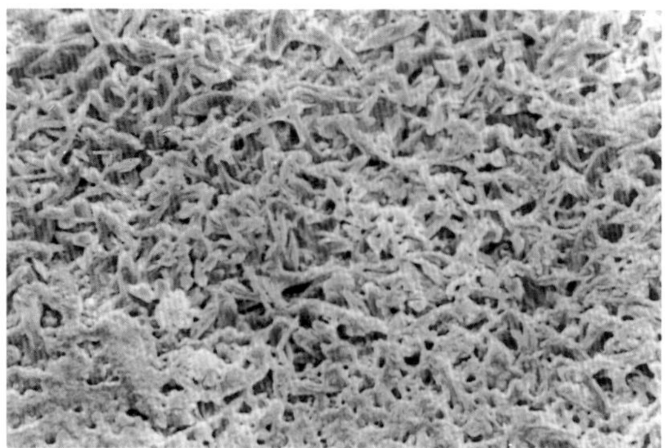

Figure 3.2

SEM of enamel surface contaminated with salt precipitates from acid allowed to remain and not washed away. (Magnification ×2030.)

give the most consistent and suitable surface for the permeation and retention of resin. Less superficial enamel is removed during etching and the reaction products are readily soluble in water (Gottlieb et al, 1982).

Phosphoric acid concentrations of less than 27% produced an insoluble by-product during the etching reaction which may be difficult to wash away. Etching with 70% phosphoric acid resulted in significantly lower tensile bond strengths of resin to enamel than those achieved with the optimum concentrations (Chow and Brown, 1973).

Etching and washing times

For some time now, the standard etching time has been set at 60 seconds, yet it is well known that it produces no better results than if a shorter etch time were used. Indeed, as far back as 1977, Brannstrom and Nordenvall had shown that etching for 15 seconds or 2 minutes gave no apparent difference in the appearance of the etch patterns. Barkmeier and co-workers (1986), in laboratory tests, found no difference in the shear strength required to remove composite resin cylinders from enamel etched for 15 or 60 seconds.

Work by Bates et al (1982) showed that a 30-second etch was practical and sufficient for bonding of resin to tooth. Scanning electron microscopy showed that no morphological differences existed in the etch pattern or character of the etched enamel rods after 30- or 60-second exposures to the acid. Ground or milled enamel surfaces produced a more uniform etch pattern than did intact surfaces, with the 60-second etch showing a greater loss of enamel substance.

Thus, it could be counterproductive to use a longer etching time because, not only does it lengthen the clinical procedure, it also increases the amount of enamel lost. Indeed, the enamel should never be over-etched because the resultant surface is too rough and prevents the free flow of the resin adhesives (Eick et al, 1972).

Clinically, the aim should be for completion of etching between 30 and 60 seconds, with timing being started after the final area of enamel is covered with acid and not at the moment of application.

Thorough washing with clean water for at least 20 seconds removes unreacted phosphoric acid and the precipitates produced during etching (Figure 3.2). It is debatable whether or not longer washing times, of up to 60 seconds, may be required to rinse off all traces of the viscous etching gel that may be trapped in the enamel micropores as a contaminant, and there is no general agreement among researchers. Clinically, a rinse time of no less than 20 seconds would be adequate, and water is best applied as a copious spray rather than as a stream, to avoid splashing.

Etching patterns

Three distinct etch patterns in enamel are discernible under the scanning electron microscope (SEM).

Type 1: Characteristic honeycomb appearance caused by preferential dissolution of the prism cores. This is the most commonly occurring pattern (see Figure 3.1b).

Type 2: Prism peripheries are preferentially removed. Due to the fact that its features resemble the natural basalt formations in County Antrim, Northern Ireland, the pattern is sometimes nicknamed the 'Giant's Causeway' (see Figure 3.1d,e).

Type 3: Characterized by a diffused surface roughening unrelated to a prism pattern (see Figure 3.1f).

All three types may be observed in the same individual, differing from surface to surface and tooth to tooth. Gwinnett (1981) reported seeing enamel devoid of etch patterns in the cervical two-thirds of the buccal surfaces of premolar and molar teeth, whilst satisfactory patterns were encountered in the incisor region of the same patient. Needless to say, it is impossible to determine with the naked eye the type of etch pattern achieved. The practitioner has to rely on a scrupulous technique and a degree of faith.

Etch patterns in deciduous enamel

Using the standard concentration of 37–50% phosphoric acid, it was thought necessary to increase the etching time to 2 min to produce comparable patterns in deciduous enamel. Initially, this apparent resistance was attributed to the presence of 'prismless enamel', but Silverstone (1978) suggested that it was more likely to be due to the lower mineral content and higher pore volume. These two factors result in the presence of larger amounts of exogenous organic material in deciduous enamel, which would otherwise show identical crystal orientation and prism arrangement as those seen in permanent enamel.

However, recent work has shown that etch patterns in deciduous enamel treated with 37% phosphoric acid for 20 seconds were no different from the patterns obtained with a 90-second etch with the proviso that the surface comprised largely of 'prismless enamel' was ground away first (Myers and Butts, 1985).

Fluoridated enamel

Fluoridated teeth are resistant to etching. This is hardly surprising because the effect of fluoride is to decrease enamel solubility. In addition, the highest concentration of fluoride is to be found in the outer surface of enamel. Generally, a longer etch time is necessary for removal of surface enamel before etching.

Long-term effects on enamel

There is no evidence that etched enamel not covered by bonding resin suffers any detrimental effects. Clinically, the etched surface is apparently restored to normal within a few days. Quantitative studies on enamel solubility rates have shown that, after 24 hours' exposure to oral fluids, a fine-grained inorganic precipitate is found to cover the etched enamel surfaces and this suggests remineralization. Etching does not render the enamel more prone to caries. Although the enamel is made more permeable by etching, there is no evidence to suggest that, given the short time the acid is in contact with the surface, any of it actually diffuses into the pulp.

Effect on dentine and pulp

In the vast majority of resin-bonded bridges, the etched enamel surface will be of prime concern. For the clinical duration of 1 or 2 minutes' etching on the enamel surface, there is little likelihood of the acid penetrating into dentine, even less into the pulp. Occasionally, however, dentine may be deliberately or inadvertently exposed as in the preparation of ledges or grooves for increasing the stability of the bridge. In such instances, should the dentine be etched? Cutting or abrading the dentine surface with burs leaves a layer of organic and inorganic detritus varying in thickness and tenacity. This so-called *dentine smear layer*

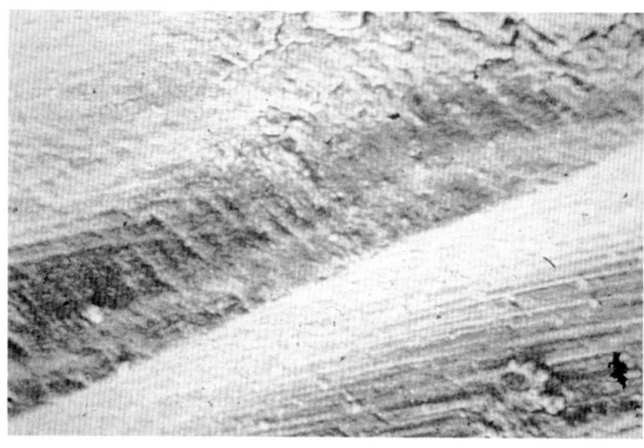

Figure 3.3.

(a) SEM of dentine smear layer. (Magnification ×1015.)

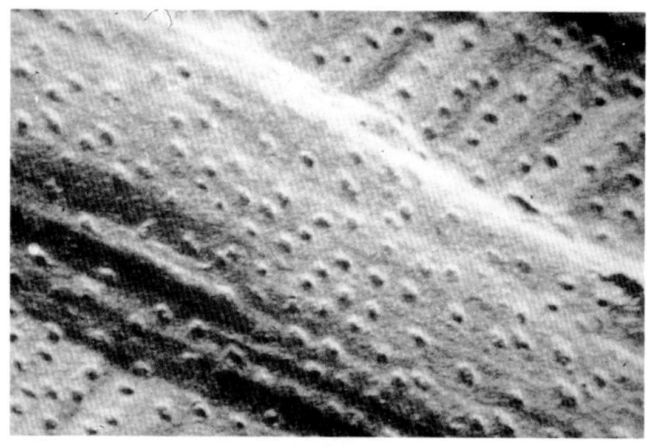

(b) Same surface after removal of smear layer with phosphoric acid solution. (Magnification ×1015.)

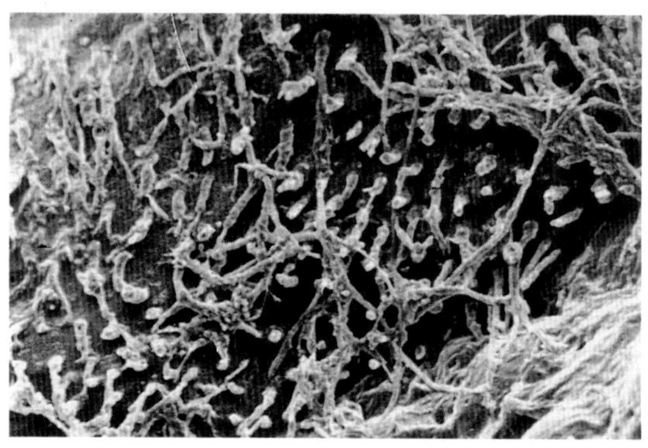

(c) SEM of fractured surface of dentine showing penetration of resin into dentinal tubules. (Magnification ×1015.)

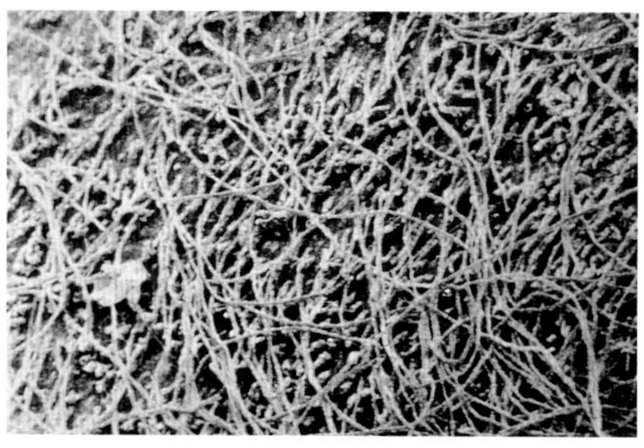

(d) The same after dissolving dentine away in formic acid showing a dense network of resin strands which have penetrated the dentinal tubules. (Magnification ×1015.)

(Figure 3.3a) presents a potential obstacle to the bonding resin. Whether or not it should be removed, indeed whether or not dentine itself should be etched, remains steeped in controversy.

Dentine, being less mineralized than enamel, does not produce the same etch pattern with phosphoric acid. Etching the cut surface removes the smear layer. Following this, there is selective removal of intratubular dentine leaving the remaining structure somewhat friable (Figure 3.3b), although the surface itself remains highly 'wettable', ie with a high surface energy, and there is usually good penetration of the resin cement (Figure 3.3c,d). A funnel-shaped widening of the tubules to a depth of 10–20 μm below the surface is created. Not only would this permit a rush of any bacteria on the surface into the dentine and eventually into the pulp to cause inflammation, but it would also promote 'moisturization' of the surface by dentinal fluid, thereby making it more difficult for the adhesive to come into intimate contact with the surface. Again, with the short clinical etching times employed, it is doubtful whether this effect is significant.

Generally, it is probably wiser not to etch dentine, but merely to dry the surface as efficiently as possible and then to use one of the special dentine bonding agents now widely available. Whatever the approach, the problem of bonding to dentine remains one of prevention of the hydrolysis of sites where forces of attraction exist between the dentine and the bonding resin.

Presence of contaminants

Exposure of tooth enamel to the oral environment results in an accumulation of a surprising amount of organic detritus on its surface. Plaque and calculus are particularly tenacious and render a high energy surface as a low energy one. A thorough brushing with mild abrasives is usually all that is required to remove superficial organic films, and calculus is readily removed with hand or ultrasonic scalers.

Water is quite a different and a much greater problem. One condensed molecular layer of water is sufficient to convert any high-energy surface into a low-energy one at room temperature. In practice, surface water is removed by blow-drying with air or by applying water-displacing agents such as butanol, acetone or ether. Unfortunately, removing the last monolayer of water is difficult, if not impossible, without destroying vital or desirable properties of the substrate surface.

Hot-air-drying of enamel after rinsing with water was shown to produce almost a 30 per cent increase in shear bond strength of resin to enamel, compared with any other drying procedure (Batchelder et al, 1987). It is possible that the hot air produces some thermal expansion within the enamel, which results in separation of the etched enamel rods. If the adhesive resin were applied immediately, it would penetrate more deeply and, as the rods contracted on cooling, the resin tags would be trapped and be difficult to dislodge.

If a liquid adhesive is unable to react with, dissolve or displace all of the surface water on the adherend, the bond will be weak when set. Conversely, if a strong bond is formed, but the adhesive has poor resistance to prolonged immersion in water, gradual deterioration of the bond will take place. It is remarkable how barnacles and other marine molluscs can maintain such strong adhesion to foreign surfaces in formidable watery environments.

The displacement of water from a surface is made easier if the adhesive is also partially miscible with water. Indeed, the bonding resins used in dentistry contain indeterminate amounts of additives, solvents, diluents or organic impurities, all of which may function as water-displacing agents, enabling the resin to achieve good wetting and adhesion.

4 Bonding resins

As the name implies, the resin-bonded bridge is attached to the surfaces of teeth with a resin cement or 'lute'. The popularity of resin-bonding techniques has produced a plethora of specialized resins, with claims of superior bond strengths as each manufacturer strives to outdo the others. It is an invidious situation, and at the present stage of development it would be foolish to attempt a single recommendation to the hard-pressed and confused practitioner. There may still appear, in due course, a cement which has such strong affinity to metal and tooth tissue that it can withstand the rigours of the oral environment, yet be kind to the tissues and easy to apply.

Ideal properties

The ideal resin for bonding metal frameworks to etched dental enamel should have the following properties:

1. Good flow and an ability to wet both etched enamel and metal surfaces.
2. Rapid and thorough setting in both aerobic and anaerobic conditions.
3. Chemical bonding with metal surfaces, the bond being unaffected by the oral environment.
4. High stiffness and strength.
5. Insoluble: properties should be unaffected by water absorption.

As indicated in Box E, there is a growing range of resins which have enough of these properties to ensure their use, although there is none that possesses all the properties. As is usual with dental materials, practitioners have developed techniques for using them despite their failings.

The available types include the following.

Dimethacrylate resins

These resins are identical to those used to form the basis of modern composites, although they may be blended in different ways. When these resins are used as the matrix for composite-filling materials, they contain between 35 and 72 per cent by volume of various types of inert, ceramic, filler particles. However, when used as a 'cement' ('luting agent' or 'lute') their filler content is nearer to 20–40 per cent by volume. One luting agent, Ultrabond (Den-Mat) is claimed to have a filler content of 65 per cent by volume.

The role of the filler in this application is to stiffen the resin both when unset and set, and to reduce the polymerization shrinkage, although at the low filler loading the contribution is not as great as it is in the filling materials.

The heavily filled restorative composite resin, as a result of its high viscosity, is generally only suitable for the bridge with a perforated design (Rochette bridge). Being translucent, these resins may not mask the 'shadowing' of the metal which is usually at the incisal third of anterior abutment teeth—an effect known as 'shine-through' (Figures 4.1 and 4.2), unless an opaquer such as titanium dioxide is first mixed in.

The 'specialized' dimethacrylate cements are lightly filled versions of the two-paste composite resin restorative materials. Chemically, they are based on either bis-GMA (bis-glycidylmethacrylate) or urethane dimethacrylate resins which are cured via the peroxide–amine reaction. When they are presented as two pastes, the peroxide initiator is in one paste and the amine activator is in the other. In some systems, the peroxide is dissolved in a solvent and this is applied as a primer to the metal and tooth surface. The paste consists of the filled resin and the amine activator.

There are also resins, such as those for bonding porcelain veneers, which may only be light-cured. But solely light-cured luting cements are a problem with metal retainers, because obviously light cannot pass through the metal. Attempts to cure the resin by transillumination through the tooth are largely ineffective, due to the distance separating the light guide from the surface of the resin and to the dissipation of light energy within the tooth substance.

Several systems now combine chemical- and light-curing agents. These are the so-called *dual curing systems*, and they combine the convenience of a 'command set' facility with the security of a room-temperature setting ability to cure the deeper layers that may not receive sufficient light intensity.

Some of these resins are available with opaquers already incorporated, whilst others have their opaquers separate—ready to be mixed in when required. As mentioned before, opaquers are required to prevent the refracted 'shadow' or 'shine-through' of the metal flange discolouring the tooth.

BOX E CEMENTS FOR RESIN-BONDED BRIDGES

Dimethacrylate cements

Paste–paste systems:	Comspan (Caulk/Dentsply)
	Epoxylite 9080 (Lee Pharmaceuticals)
	Maryland Bridge Cementation Kit (Den-Mat)
	Maryland Bridge Cement (Teledyne Getz)
	Nimetic Grip (ESPE)
Paste–primer systems:	Duralingual Bonded Bridge Cement (Unitek)
	Maryland Bridge Cement (Lee Pharmaceuticals)
Dual-curing systems:	Dual Cement (Ivoclar/Vivadent)
	Duo-Cure (Terec)
	Microfill Pontic C (Kultzer)
	Ultra Bond (Den-Mat)

Chemically adhesive cements

Bis-GMA with active phosphate ester:
- ABC Cement (Ivoclar/Vivadent)
- Clearfil New Bond (Kuraray)
- Panavia-EX (Kuraray)

Bipolyester with zinc oxide:
- F-21 (Voco)

Epoxy resin, acrylic modified:
- Lee Metal Primer (Lee Pharmaceuticals)

4-META, methyl methacrylate:
- Super-Bond C&B (Sun Medical)

Methacrylate terpolymer:
- Gold Link 2 (Den-Mat)

Glass-ionomer, methacrylate:
- Geristore (Den-Mat)

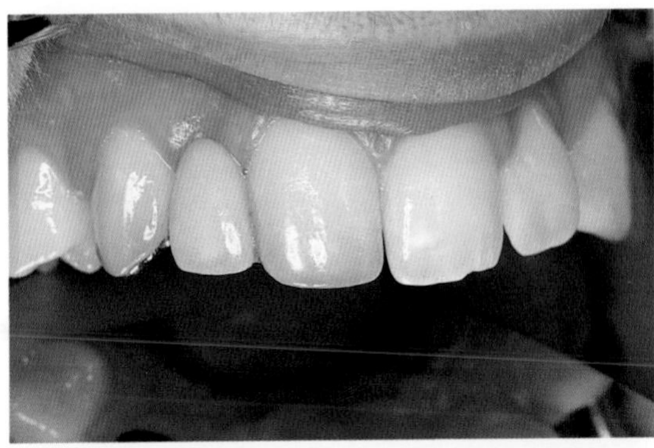

Figure 4.1

Shadow of metal showing through translucent incisal enamel in upper right central incisor. This is caused by a lack of opaquers in the resin cement and is often referred to as the 'shine-through' effect.

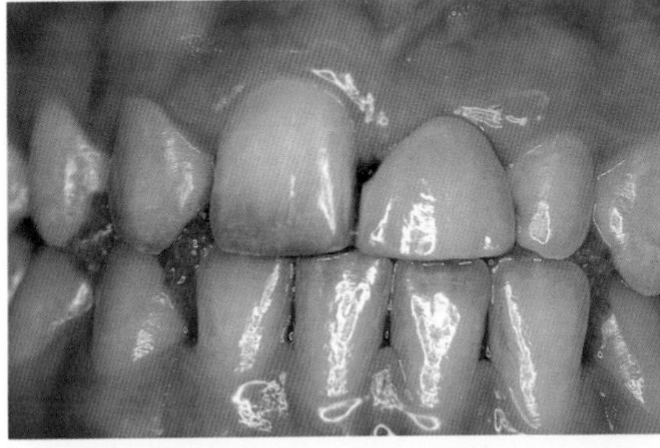

Figure 4.2

(a) Another example of 'shine-through' affecting the upper right central incisor.

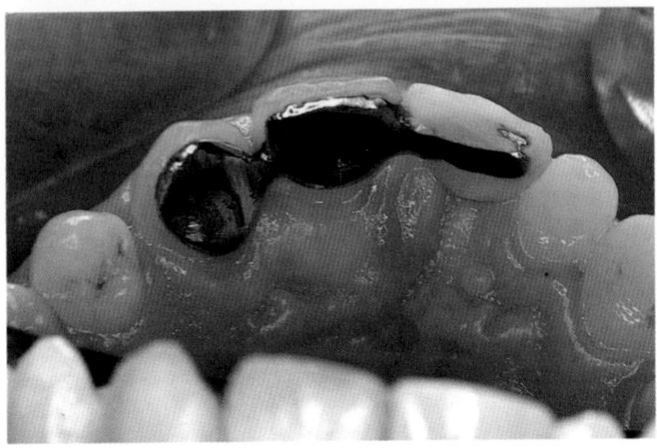

(b) Lingual view of the same case.

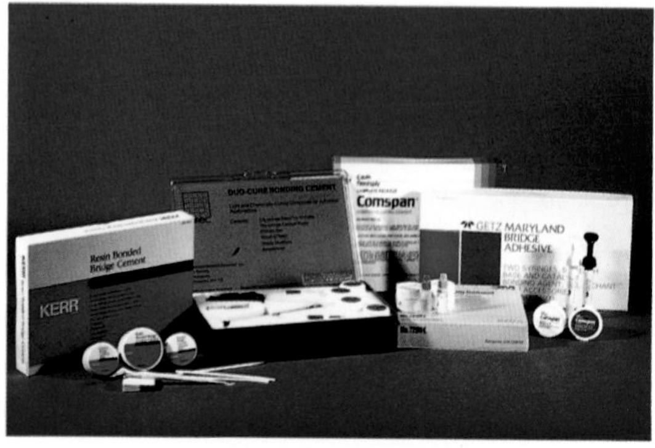

Figure 4.3

A selection of commercial brands of dimethacrylate resin cements marketed specifically for resin-bonded bridges. Most contain an opaquer.

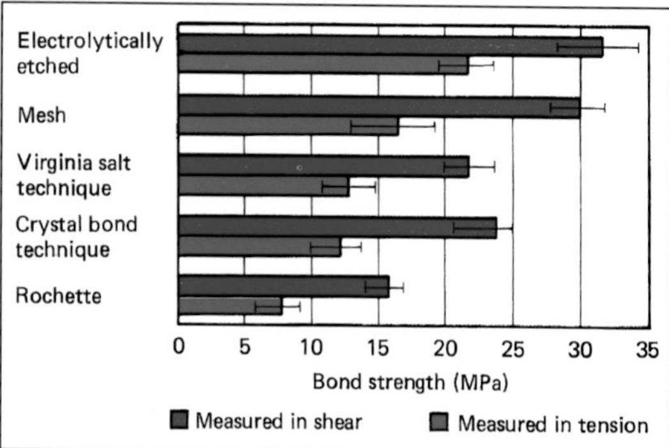

Figure 4.4

Bar graph showing the relative bond strengths tested in shear and in tension of Comspan (Caulk/Dentsply) resin bonded to a nickel–chromium alloy with surface features produced by various techniques.

All examples of these resins possess high flow and low film thickness enabling penetration into the etch pits and into and around any cast-in surface features. When efficiently retained, the strength of the bond between the resin and the metal surface is limited by the strength of the resin itself and, as seen in Figure 2.20b, failure occurs cohesively within the cement. A selection of commercially available resins is shown in Figure 4.3.

Average bond-strength values of a representative dimethacrylate resin, Comspan (Caulk-Dentsply), when applied to various types of retentive forms, are illustrated in Figure 4.4.

Intermediary resins

A number of resin systems designed to help the dimethacrylate resin cements bond to either precious or base-metal alloys are less satisfactory in their ability to form a strong and permanent adhesive bond to the metal. These resin systems are in essence resin-based primers. They include the Lee Metal Primer and Gold Link. The Lee Metal Primer is an epoxy resin and heat-curing agent which contains white titanium dioxide as an opacification medium. It is diluted with a solvent to make it easy to apply. In use, it is applied in a thin layer to either an etched or sandblasted surface, which must be clean, dry and free from any oily contaminants. The primer is then baked at 185°C for exactly 10 minutes—no more and no less. A thin layer of a traditional amine–peroxide curing methyl methacrylate is added to the cool surface and this is also baked at 185°C—this time for an hour. The treated framework can then be cemented using one of the dimethacrylate resins. This should be carried out within 14 days of the production of the baked resin sandwich.

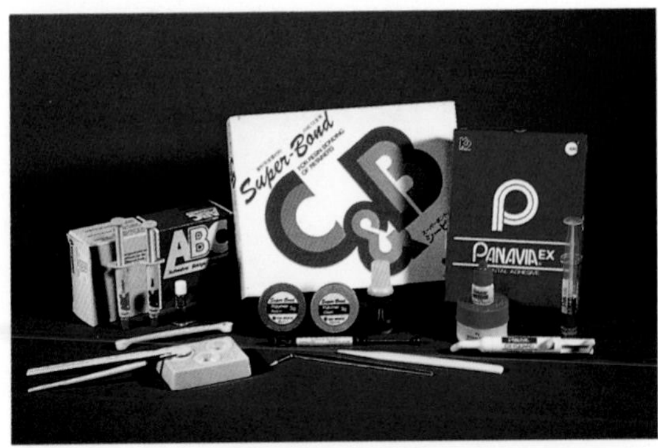

Figure 4.5

A selection of commercial brands of so-called chemically adhesive 'bifunctional' resins.

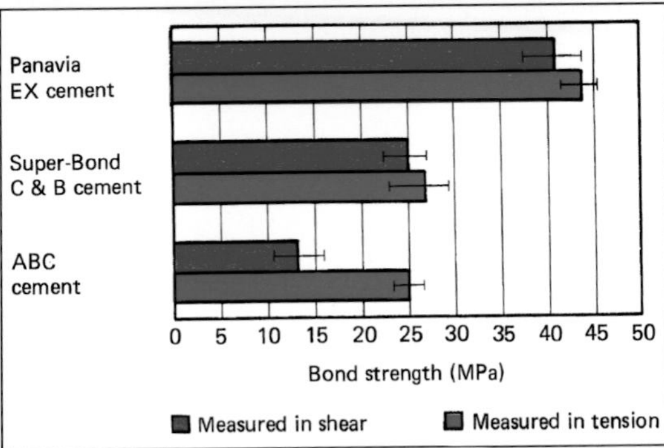

Figure 4.6

Bar graph showing the relative shear and tensile bond strengths of three commercial brands of chemically adhesive cements bonded to sandblasted NP2 alloy.

The Gold Link system. utilizes a light-curing dimethacrylate resin which contains an opacifying pigment that consequently has to be cured for 90 seconds.

Shear bond strength for both systems, on unetched, primed, non-precious metal and using a dimethacrylate luting resin, is reputed to be in the region of 12–13 MPa.

Chemically adhesive cements

Another approach to utilizing the whole of the fitting surface in the formation of a retentive bond is to use a resin that inherently forms a bond to the metal. A number of these resins have been developed over the last few years, mainly in Japan (Figure 4.5). The resins which have shown the most promise utilize 'bifunctional' or 'dual affinity' compounds which form chemical bonds with clean, sandblasted metal surfaces at one end and with lightly filled resins containing methacrylate groups at the other.

Materials currently available include methacrylate resins with metal-seeking ends which are based on either derivatives of alkyl phosphonic acid, modified phosphate esters, trimellitic acid or its anhydride (4-META). The resin-seeking ends contain vinyl double bonds. These adhesives are attracted to the passive oxide film found on chromium-containing alloys, although the formation of an excessively thick layer of oxide often produces an inferior bond. Attempts have been made to promote bonding to precious metal alloys by plating them with tin and then forming an oxide layer to which the bifunctional resins will be attracted (Wada, 1986). Results appear to be promising, as does sandblasting with 50 µm alumina followed by a heating cycle which probably

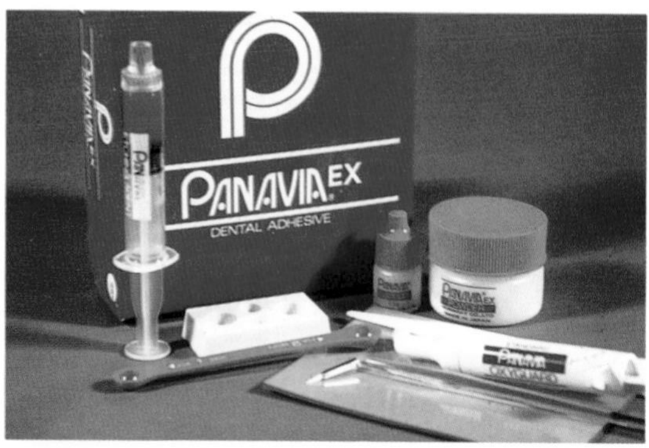

Figure 4.7

(a) Panavia EX (Kuraray)—a popular chemically adhesive cement.

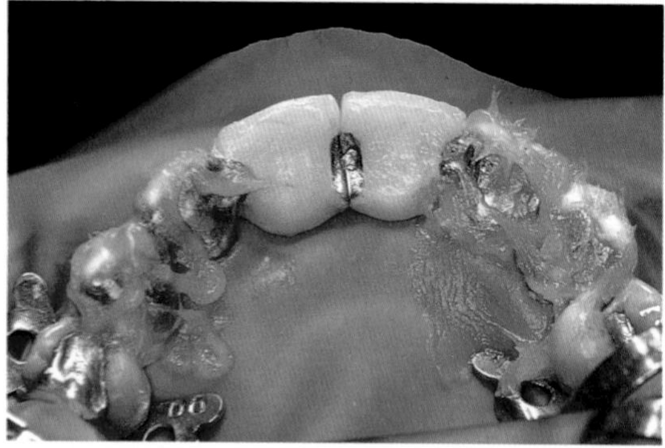

(b) Exclusion of air from the surface of the resin is necessary for it to set, and this is achieved by applying the blue 'grease' (Oxyguard) supplied by the manufacturer.

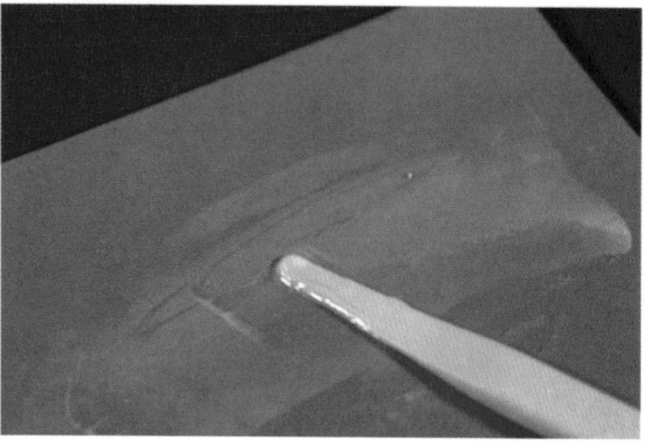

(c) The cement should be spread thinly over the pad during mixing of the powder and liquid. This exposes the cement film to air and will prevent premature setting.

causes some of the alumina to be retained within the metal surface.

Figure 4.6 shows the comparative bond strengths, under certain laboratory conditions, of three commercial, dual-affinity, resin cements to sandblasted, non-precious metal surfaces (Atta et al, 1990). These show very similar values in both tension and shear and, in the case of Panavia EX (Figure 4.7a), which contains a phenyl phosphate ester, the values are considerably higher than any values obtained with resins bonded to either cast-in or etched surfaces.

Resins based on either methyl methacrylate, bis-GMA or urethane dimethacrylate are used to link bifunctional metal primers with the etched enamel. Several contain tributylborane for the promotion of adhesion to tooth structure and the reduction of the amount of air inhibition shown by these resins. Even so, exclusion of air is necessary to promote complete polymerization and, in one product, Panavia EX, this is achieved by covering the resin at the margins of the metal flange with a thick 'grease' to exclude air from the surface (Figure 4.7b).

On the whole, these resins are used to bond *flat*, sandblasted metal surfaces, ie those without cast-in or etched features. Particularly with the latter, weak bonds may be formed due to the presence of air in the etch pits which prevents setting of the resin (Atta et al, 1988). Also, with an anaerobic setting cement such as Panavia EX, it is essential that puddles are not formed on the mixing pad because the lower layers, consequent on being excluded from air, may set prematurely. Rather, the mixing technique is to spread the cement out as thinly as possible on the pad (Figure 4.7c), only finally bringing the mass into a pool to be scooped up into the flange. Panavia EX also has a recommended mixing time of 1 minute, and this must be strictly observed, preferably with the aid of a stopwatch or electronic timer.

Recently, a material with the putative ability to bond aggressively to tooth tissue, porcelain and metal has been introduced. This material, Geristore (Den-Mat Corp.), is a small particle, glass-ionomer-based composite resin with a facility for 'dual-curing'—that is, command setting via a light source as well as auto-curing via a chemical reaction. Other features include radiopacity, hydrophilic properties and a capacity for leaching fluoride ions. Although no long-term trials have yet been published, the material exemplifies the trend among dental manufacturers to seek the all-purpose resin.

Finally, whatever the choice of resin adhesive, the fundamental rule is always that surfaces to be bonded must be scrupulously clean and free from contamination with saliva, oil and dirt, and dental plaque. Both operator and assistant must be familiar with the manufacturer's instructions. It is surprising how many mishaps occur through lack of care in the mixing and handling of the cement.

5 Bridge design

Introduction

It is difficult to lay down an infallible prescription for selecting a particular bridge design. In designing and planning conventional bridges, Smith (1990) bemoaned the fact that bridge design was 'complex, poorly researched and dominated by personal opinions derived from clinical experience, or lack of it'. With the relatively novel, yet simple, technique of resin-bonded bridges, design concepts have been in a continual state of evolution and mutation since the late Michael Buonocore first promulgated the acid-etch technique over a quarter of a century ago. However, recently there appears to be an encouraging rise in the number of published long-term clinical trials from which much understanding of the behaviour of these bridges can be gleaned.

In the final analysis, the practitioner is dependent on the probity and perspicacity of the clinical investigator, and the guidelines offered in this chapter are based on the findings of several such investigators. Whether or not these criteria will remain valid for the next decade is conjectural. The oft-quoted philosopher, Heraclitus (about 500 BC) may be enlisted to give assurance that 'nothing is permanent but change'.

Types of bridges

As for conventional bridges, resin-bonded bridges may be considered according to the five basic types given below.

Fixed–fixed

All the components of the bridge are rigidly connected. This is the most common type of resin-bonded bridge (Figure 5.1).

Fixed–movable

The bridge is in two parts, locked or keyed together by a non-rigid connector or attachment (Figure 5.2). This attachment, which may be either prefabricated or laboratory-made, permits movement of the two parts relative to each other in only one plane, usually the vertical. The use of movable joints in resin-bonded bridges will be discussed in the following sections.

Cantilever

The pontic is supported at only one end, ie 'cantilevered' from one side of the abutment tooth which may be either mesial or distal to the pontic (Figures 5.3 and 5.4). The main indication for a cantilevered bridge is in situations where the teeth on one side or the other of the pontic are unsuitable as abutments either due to the poor quality of the enamel for bonding or because there are prevailing cosmetic reasons, such as an unfavourable angulation of an abutment tooth or the presence of a diastema. As a consequence of the pontic being held at only one end, the stress on the retainer is far greater than in a fixed–fixed or fixed–movable type. This design is therefore not recommended in areas of high occlusal stress. Its main use is in the replacement of an upper lateral incisor where the upper canine happens to be a particularly suitable abutment tooth. Cantilever bridges are also the easiest to clean from the patient's point of view.

Spring cantilever

This bridge is restricted to the upper anterior region where the presence of gaps (diastemas) or unsuitable (ie crowned) abutment teeth are present

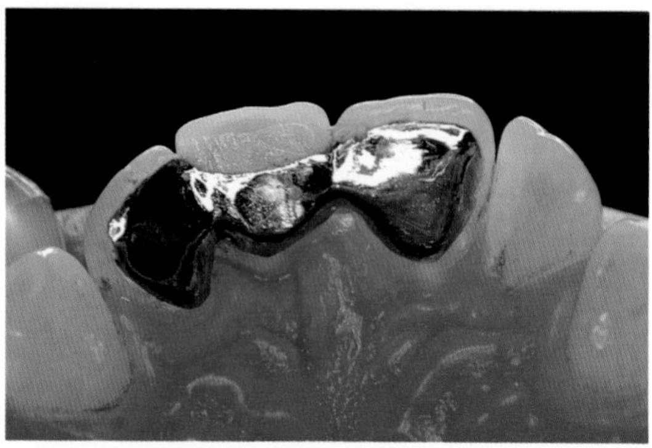

Figure 5.1

Examples of the fixed–fixed design of resin-bonded bridge replacement in (a) upper right central incisor,

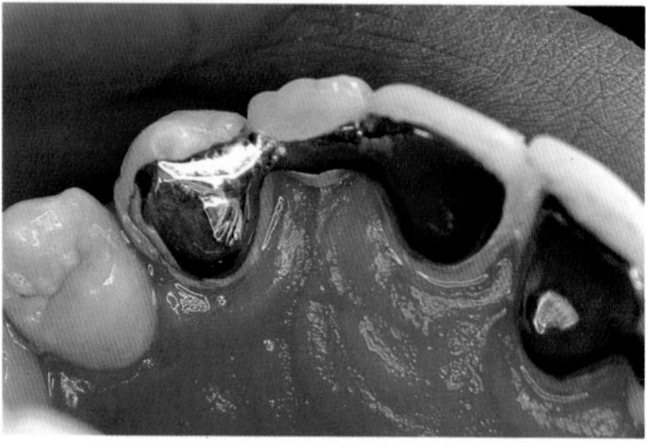

(b) upper right lateral incisor,

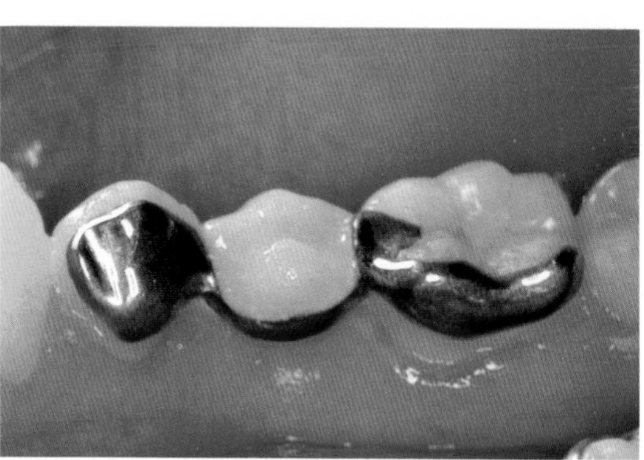

(c) lower right second premolar.

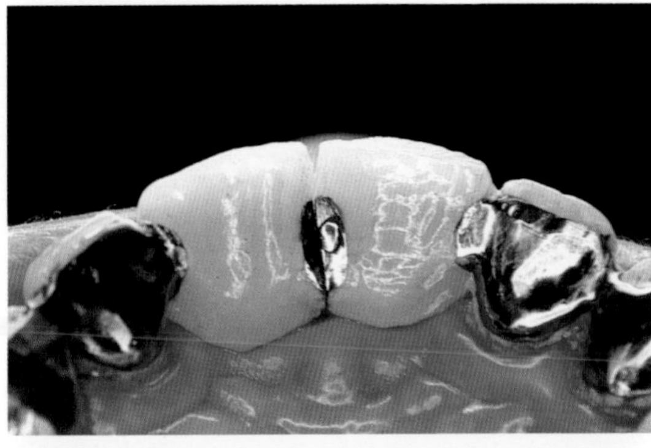

Figure 5.2

Example of a fixed–movable design. The non-rigid or movable attachment is located between the two central incisor pontics.

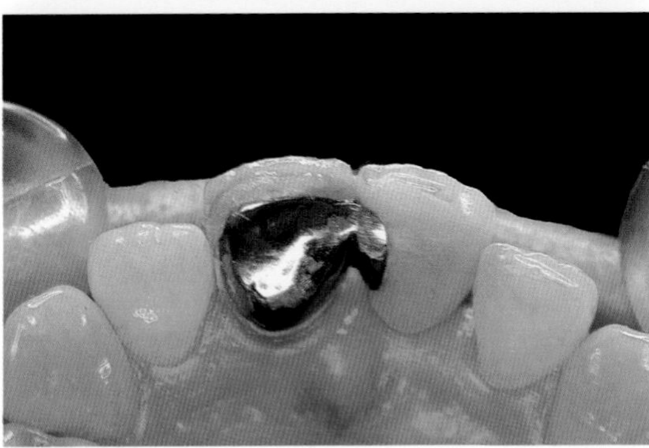

Figure 5.3

Example of a cantilever design. The upper left central incisor pontic is retained solely by the upper right central incisor.

(Figure 5.5). Only one pontic can be supported and is connected to a distant abutment tooth or teeth by a fairly long, slightly flexible bar which, in turn, rests on and is supported by the compressible soft tissue of the palate. The 'springiness' of the bar acts as a 'shock absorber' and attenuates excessive leverage forces on the abutment tooth or teeth.

Hybrid

This is a combination of a conventional crown at one end and a resin-bonded retainer at the other end of the pontic (Figures 5.6–5.8). The joints may be either 'fixed' or 'movable'. Generally, in the fixed–fixed design, the differences in retentive modes between the conventional and resin-bonded units may place the latter at greater risk of coming loose if the bridge is subjected to undue stresses.

Factors in resin-bonded bridge design

A number of clinical surveys have shown that the failure rate of resin-bonded bridges varies from nil to as high a figure as 50 per cent or more (Hamada et al, 1985; Tay, 1986; Kellett, 1987; Clyde and Boyd, 1988; Williams et al, 1989; Creugers et al, 1990).

A recent survey by Hussey et al (1991) bears this out. These authors reviewed 400 resin-bonded bridges of several types over a period of

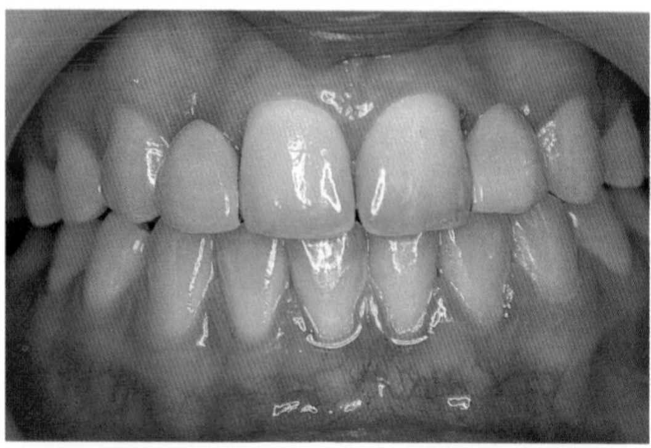

Figure 5.4

A pair of cantilever resin-bonded bridges replacing upper left and right lateral incisors: (a) labial view;

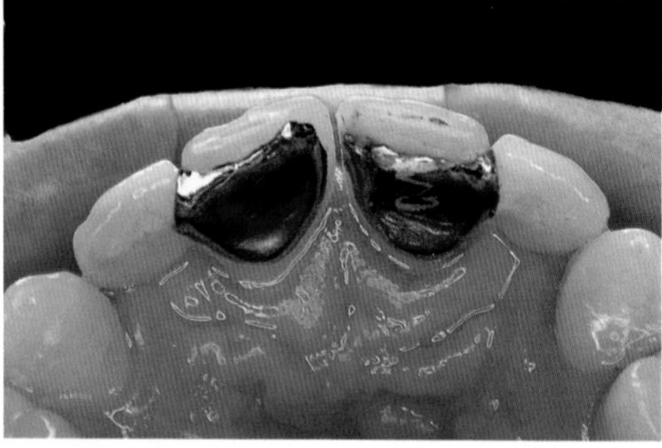

(b) lingual view.

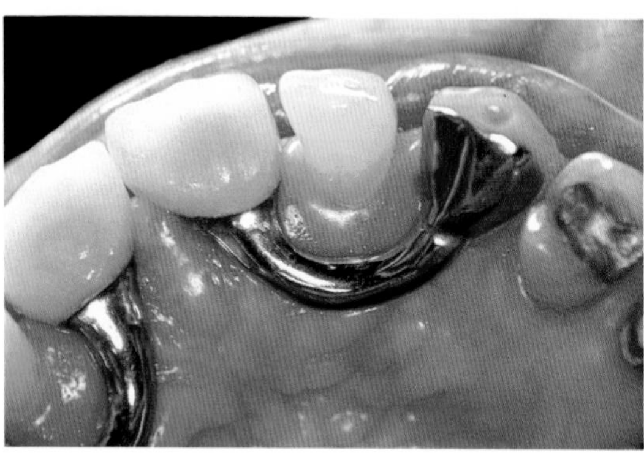

Figure 5.5

Two spring cantilever bridges replacing the upper central incisors. Support and retention of each pontic comes via a 'spring' bar and retainer on the canine. The bar itself is supported by the compressible mucosa of the palate. (Courtesy of Dr D.L. Hussey.)

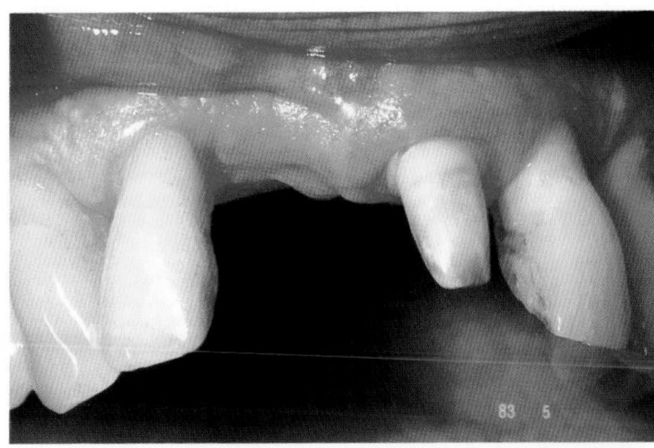

Figure 5.6

Hybrid design: (a) conventional jacket crown preparation on the upper left central incisor;

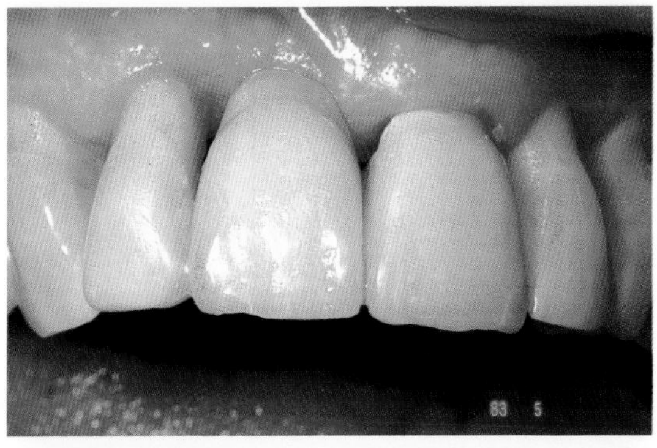

(b) bridge in place;

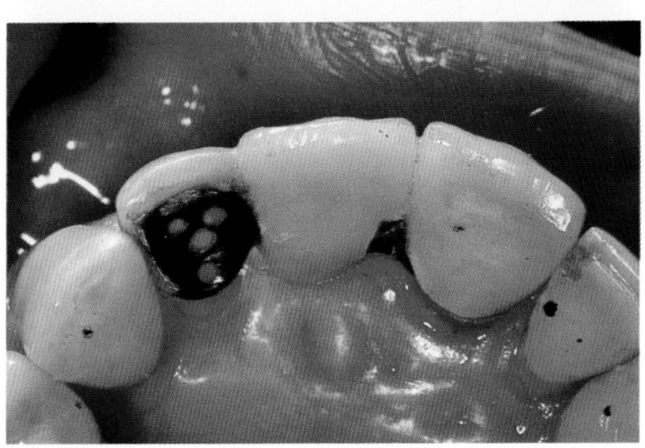

(c) lingual view showing conventional jacket crown retainer on the upper left central incisor and resin-bonded retainer (perforated type) on the upper right lateral incisor. (Courtesy of Mr R. Mitzman.)

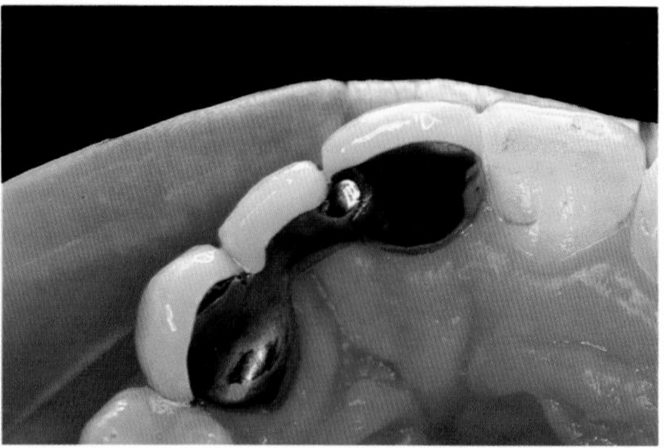

Figure 5.7

Hybrid design replacing upper right lateral incisor with conventional crown retainer on the upper right canine and resin-bonded retainer with non-rigid attachment on the upper right central incisor.

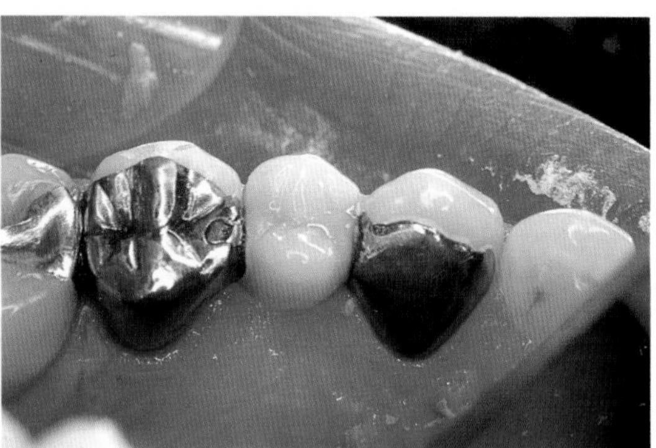

Figure 5.8

Hybrid design replacing upper right first premolar with conventional crown bearing a non-rigid attachment on the upper right second premolar and with a resin-bonded retainer on the canine. (Courtesy of Dr D.L. Hussey.)

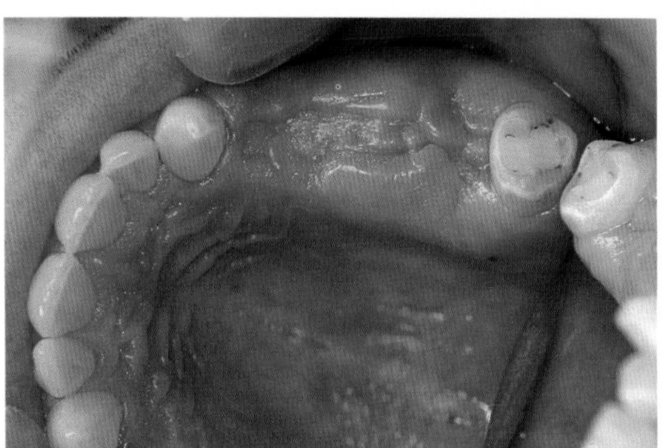

Figure 5.9

Hybrid design replacing upper left premolars and molar. (a) The upper left canine has a malformed crown which was prepared to receive a porcelain veneer on the labial aspect, with a metal brace resting on a rest seat prepared on the palatal aspect. The last molar was prepared minimally to receive an etched porcelain occlusal onlay.

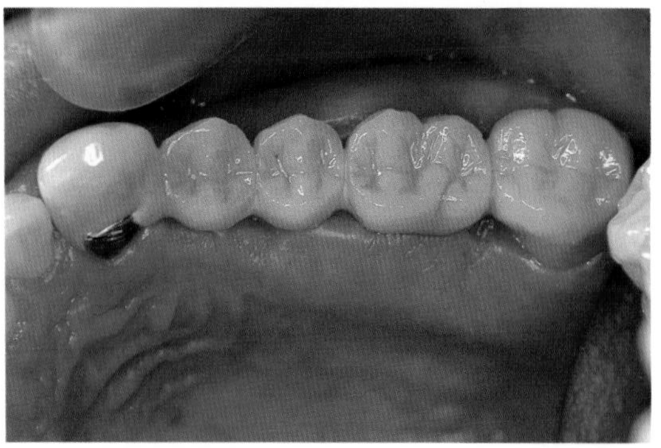

(b) The final bridge in place. Incorporated in the design is a subframe of Ni–Cr–Be alloy that runs the length of the bridge and supports the porcelain onlay on the last molar tooth through the porcelain pontics and onto the palatal brace on the canine. The metal surfaces in contact with the tooth have been etched in the usual manner. Greater support could have been achieved if the palatal brace had covered the whole of the palatal surface. (Courtesy of Dr E. Lynch.)

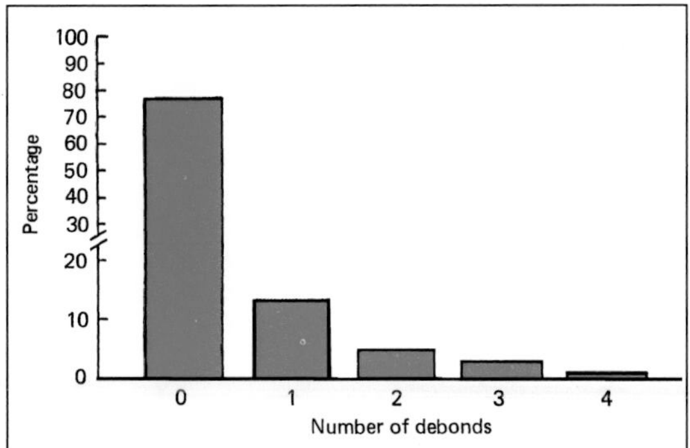

Figure 5.10.

Bar graphs of clinical studies of Maryland resin-bonded bridges (see text). (a) This illustrates the clinical performance of anterior and posterior resin-bonded bridges—the combined results. (After Hussey et al, 1991.).

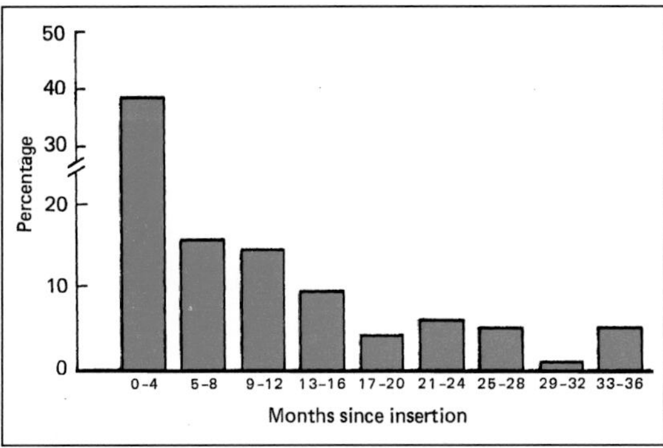

(b) Frequency of debonds. The figures indicate months to the occurrence of the first debond. (After Hussey et al, 1991.)

3.4 years and found, for example, that with both anterior and posterior Maryland bridges taken as a whole, about 78 per cent of bridges remained intact throughout (Figure 5.10a): about 13 per cent suffered a single debond, 5 per cent had two debond episodes, but 1 per cent encountered four debonds. Thirty-nine per cent of the first debonds usually occurred within 4 months of placement with a total of 70 per cent of bridges becoming detached within the first year (Figure 5.10b). Posterior bridges seemed to have a slight edge over anterior bridges in resisting debonding (Figure 5.10c), and this is probably due to the fact that the morphological features of, say, a molar tooth present greater potential for retentive and stable designs than a slim incisor tooth.

There is also good evidence that cantilever bridges are reliable in the mouth (Tay and Shaw, 1979; Hopkins, 1981; Shaw and Tay, 1982; Tay, 1987; Clyde and Boyd, 1988). Hussey et al (1991) have shown that these bridges may have a success rate of 85 per cent when compared with other designs of Maryland bridges (Figure 5.10d).

From the surveys looked at, it can be deduced that the average would appear to be around 20 per cent over periods of 2–6 years (Tay, 1986). This compares unfavourably with surveys of conventional bridges which tend to hover around the 2–7 per cent figure over periods of 5–10 years (Roberts, 1970; Reuter and Brose, 1984; Karlsson, 1986).

The Rochette bridge (perforated retainer) in particular has been singled out for censure, with the 'macromechanical' mode of retention of the perforations being cited as the major drawback. As mentioned previously, retention is confined to the immediate region of each perforation; occlusal stresses are effectively concentrated on

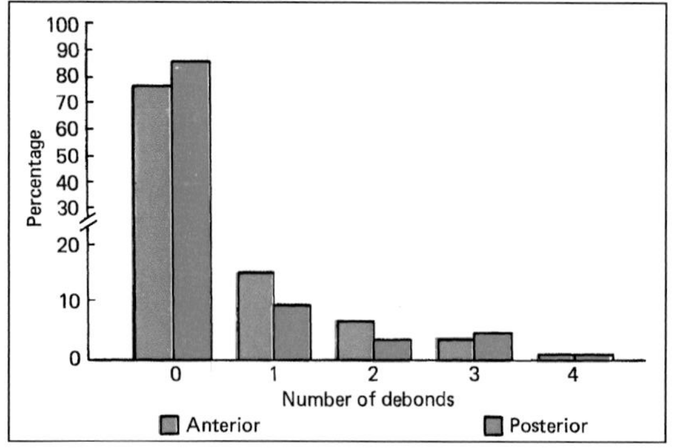

(c) Comparison between anterior and posterior bridges. (After Hussey et al, 1991.)

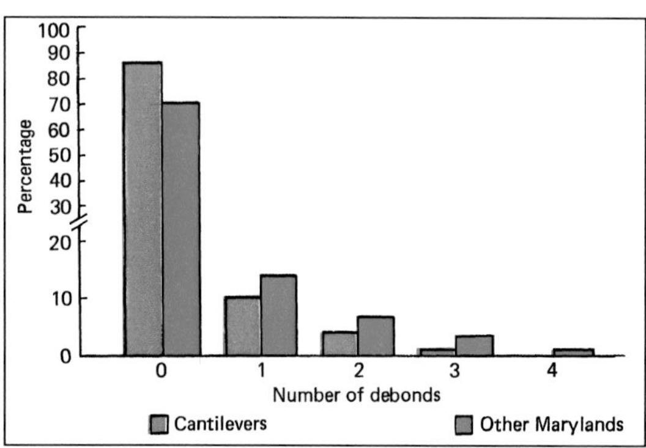

(d) The success rate of cantilever bridges. (After Hussey et al, 1991.)

the few narrow protrusions of resin. Furthermore, the exposed resin may be prone to abrasive wear or long-term hydrolytic breakdown at the filler–matrix interface. Eventually, micro-leakage and bond failure (or 'debond', in the adhesive chemists' parlance) would occur. However, Figure 5.11 illustrates a case of extensive wear of the flanges of two cantilevered Rochette bridges after 5 years in the mouth without deterioration of the bond.

Although it is believed that a non-perforated design would enhance the durability of the restoration, recent surveys have shown that even non-perforated retainers are subject to high failure rates of around 30 per cent (Williams et al, 1989), and therefore other factors must be considered. These include:

1 The quality of the tooth enamel and the thoroughness of the etching procedure.
2 The design of the retainer (flange).
3 The design of the pontic.
4 The luting resin used.

Thus, the correct bridge design is an important factor in clinical success, and should be influenced not so much by the mode of retention (which, in a way, is determined by the facilities available) but by the considerations of the quality of the abutment teeth, cosmetic factors ('aesthetics') and stability or resistance of the bridge to displacing forces. Therefore, a thorough assessment of the patient's mouth, assisted by good radiographs and study models, is essential. Alleviation of displacing or debonding stresses is crucial, and a good design

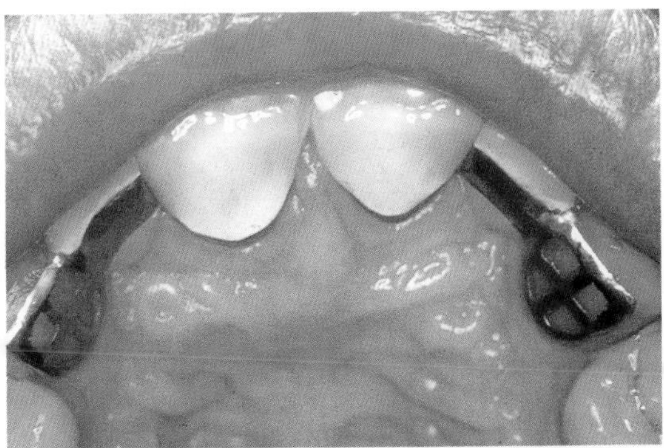

Figure 5.11

An example of two Rochette cantilever bridges which have lasted well over 8 years in spite of gross wear on the retainers. (a) Lingual view at placement (note that the colour of the transparency has not withstood the passage of time).

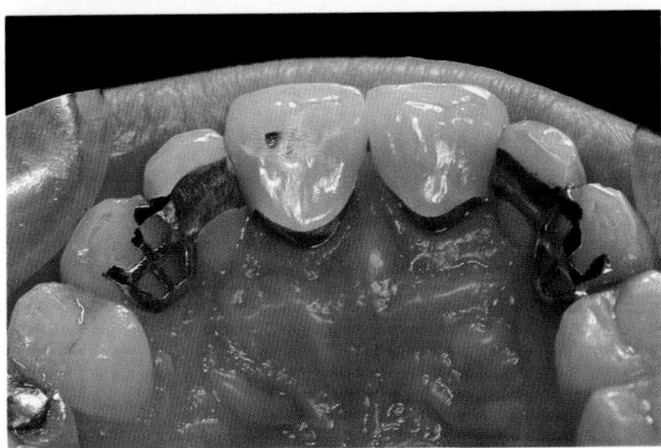

(b) Appearance at a recent recall. Note the wear on the perforated retainers and on the metal–ceramic crown of the upper right central incisor.

should display features that will resist these forces both laterally and occlusally (or gingivally).

Retainer design

A stable and durable bridge may be devised by: having a strong and rigid framework; ensuring maximum coverage of retainer over the abutment teeth to ensure sufficient retention and resistance form; using movable joints (stress-breakers).

Rigid framework

Base metal (or non-precious metal) alloys are most suitable for resin-bonded bridges. When cast, they are strong, rigid and resistant to wear even in thin sections. Certainly, if perforated retainers are to be used, base metal alloys are obligatory. As a rule, with base metal alloys, 0.3 mm is given as the minimum thickness of metal required where it is overlaid with porcelain, in order to contain the flexural stress fractures of porcelain.

Photoelastic stress analysis of resin-bonded bridges has shown that high stresses are developed within the retainer, especially on the lingual aspect (Caputo et al, 1986). These stresses are reduced by thickening the retainer and extending it into the approximal region. Thus, the recommended minimum thickness of a retainer is given as 0.6 mm at the lingual and approximal aspects, but over the occlusal contact areas the metal needs only to be 0.1-mm thick.

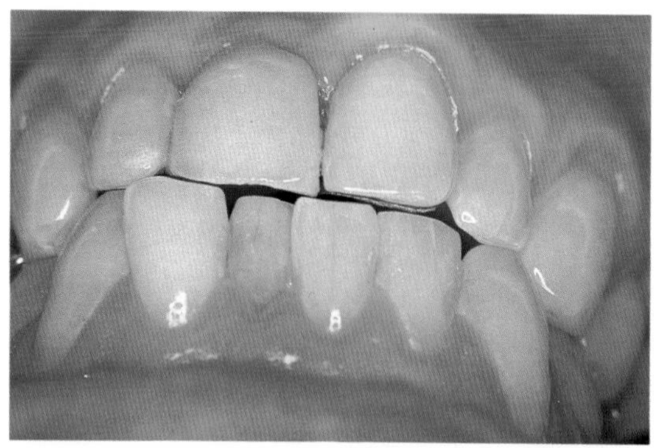

Figure 5.12

The 'inlay' effect on a four-unit resin-bonded bridge replacing the upper right central incisor (see text). (a) Protrusive relationship showing how stresses on the pontic and abutment may contribute to the loosening of the upper left central incisor flange;

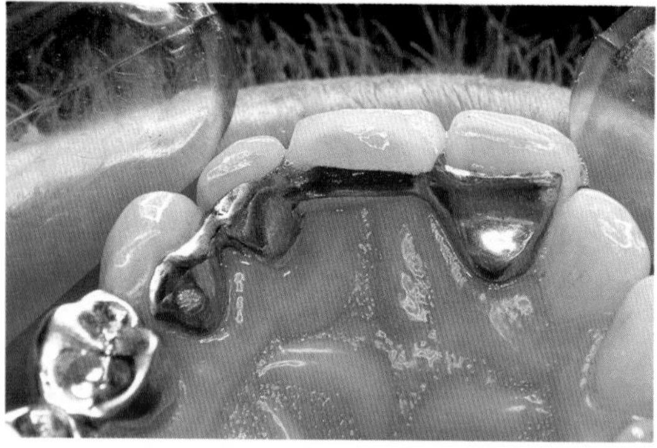

(b) lingual view;

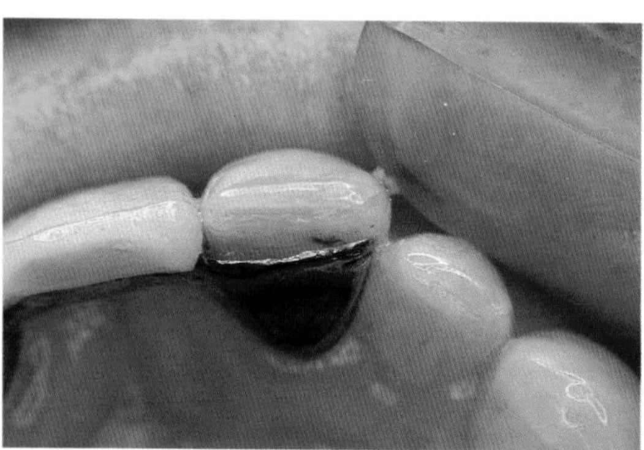

(c) lingual view close-up showing the detached (debonded) flange.

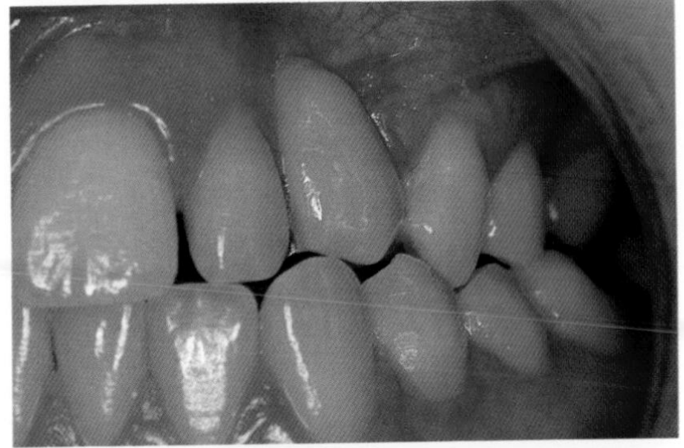

a

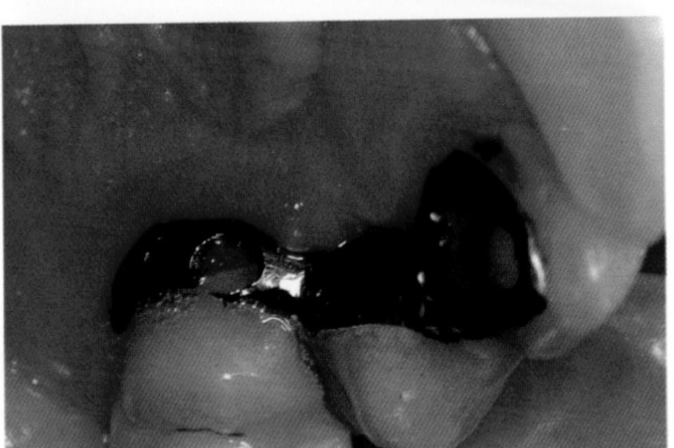

b

Figure 5.13 (a, b)

Resin-bonded bridge replacing upper left canine. (a) Lateral stresses on the canine pontic, aggravated by lack of adequate occlusal support, have led to debonding of the skimpy retainers and impaction of the pontic into the mucosa in (b).

Maximum coverage

At this point in the history of resin-bonded bridges, there is insufficient information to dictate the minimum surface area of retainer coverage conducive to maximum bonding. Nevertheless, it is a simple precept that the greater the area of abutment tooth covered, the greater the retention. The extent of a retainer may be considered as (1) the outline form and (2) the physiological form.

Outline form

The actual outline of the flange is governed by the following:

1 The length of pontic span.
2 Occlusal contacts.
3 Resistance and retention.
4 Presence of existing restorations.

Length of pontic span

In conventional bridgework, it is often stated that, the longer the span of a bridge, the greater the stress placed on the abutment teeth and bridge retainers. The problem seems to be exacerbated during mastication of a bolus of food. With no food in the mouth, closure in the intercuspal position (centric closure)* tends to distribute forces along all the occlusal surfaces of the arch and

* Intercuspal position (ICP): the mandibulomaxillary relationships in which the cusps and sulci of the mandibular and maxillary teeth mesh together tightly. This is usually the most cranial position of the mandible.

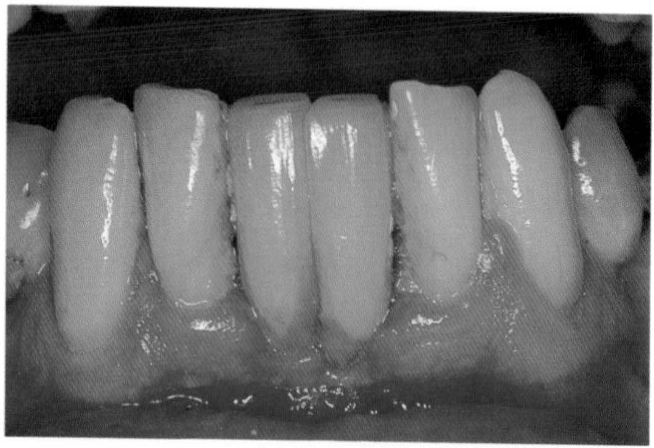

Figure 5.14

Poor pontic design has reduced or obliterated the embrasure spaces making it difficult for the patient to keep the area clean. (a) Labial view.

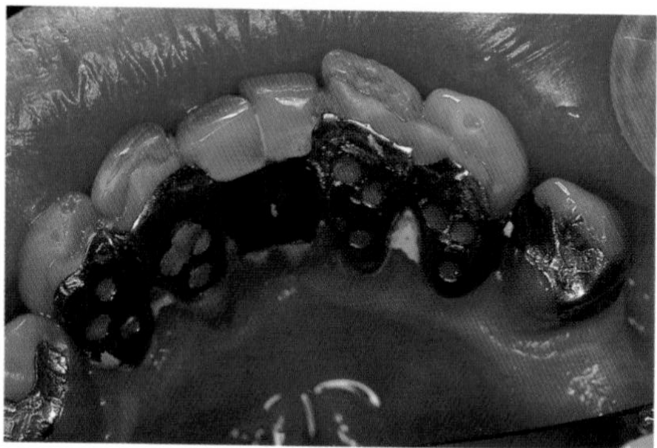

(b) Lingual view showing accumulation of calculus under the pontic and flanges.

therefore poses only slight problems of flexure of the bridge. However, if a bolus of food is positioned between the pontic of a long span bridge and the opposing occlusal surfaces, the effect may be quite unexpected because the opposing occlusal contacts have not yet 'come into play'. All the force would be directed onto the pontic span, setting up stresses which the retainers and/or abutment teeth may not be able to withstand.

A formula was developed by Ante (1926), now known as 'Ante's law', which states that the root surface area of the abutment teeth should equal or surpass the root surface area of the tooth/teeth to be replaced. It is tempting to paraphrase this rule to apply to the available bonding surfaces of the abutment teeth in resin-bonded bridges. But because Ante's law itself has been criticized for lack of scientific evidence, and not least because it does not give the full picture of the interplay of factors, the use of multiple retainers in resin-bonded bridges must also be said to be empirical. Whilst the premise that the greater the surface covered, the stronger the retention applies well to the individual abutment tooth, the same cannot be assumed for multiple retainers. The long-span bridge with its multiple retainers connects a number of abutment teeth rigidly, so that in effect they all function as one unit without deference to the intrinsic physiological movement of each abutment tooth. Furthermore, unless there is complete coverage of the occlusal planes by the retainer, the exposed areas of the abutment teeth may be subjected to normal occlusal loading which could stress the resin–metal or resin–tooth bond by virtue of the deflective forces imposed (Figures 5.12 and 5.13). The situation is

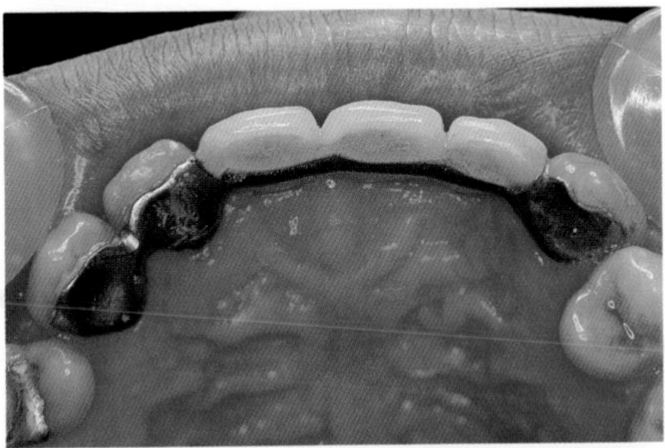

a

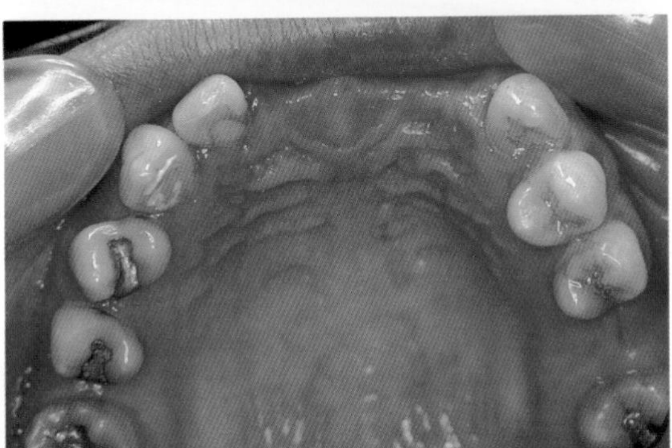

b

Figure 5.15 (a, b)

In long-span, anterior resin-bonded bridges, the curvature of the dental arch may pose problems due to the difficulty in keeping the pontics within the confines of the abutments.

not dissimilar to that occurring in a conventional fixed–fixed bridge with cast inlays as retainers. Due to the fact that the inlay is held rigidly by the bridge, occlusal loading of an uncovered cusp, for example, may depress the tooth and 'bite it away' from the inlay. Also, it must be remembered that gaining maximum coverage by increasing the number of retainers may be counterproductive where the natural tooth embrasures are obliterated by the metal framework, making it impossible for the patient to clean between the teeth (Figure 5.14).

In the anterior region, the curvature of the arch imposes more stresses on the bridge because the pontics cannot be kept within the confines of the interabutment axis (Figure 5.15).

The most difficult tooth to replace is the maxillary canine which often lies outside this axis. A further complication is that the lateral incisor is most unsuitable as an abutment tooth due to the comparatively small bonding surface. A cantilever bridge with conjoined first and second premolar (bicuspid) retainers may be feasible *provided* no occlusal loading from canine guidance is present (Figure 5.16). If a canine and a premolar are missing, then it is best if they are replaced by a conventional bridge or removable partial denture.

Occlusal contacts

Due to the 'inlay effect' mentioned previously, it may be desirable to cover the whole occluding surface of an abutment tooth with the flange in the manner of a conventional three-quarter crown. However, this is only feasible where there are no occlusal contacts present, ie in 'open-bite'

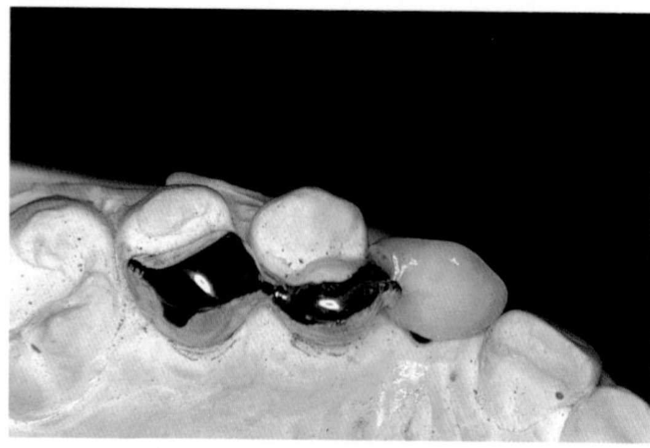

Figure 5.16

Cantilever bridge replacing upper right canine. (a) Working model showing conjoined retainers on the upper first right and second premolars. Note the extent of coverage of the retainers.

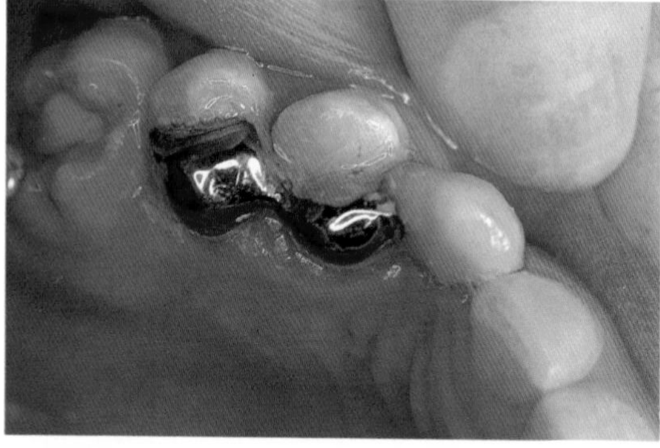

(b) The bridge in the mouth.

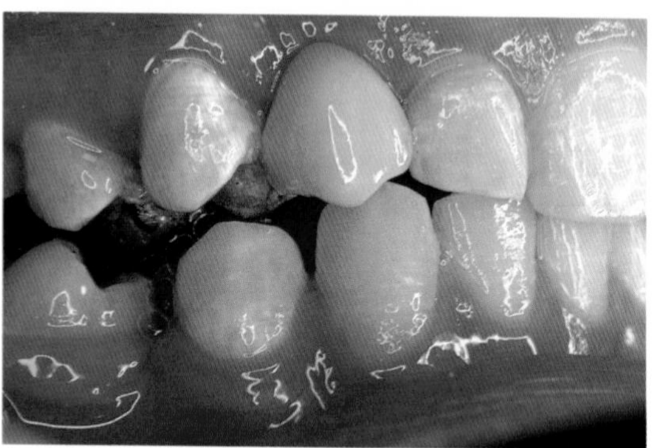

(c) Labial view of the same showing absence of non-working side interferences in spite of coverage of lingual cusps.

situations. With no gross reduction of the abutment teeth in resin-bonded bridges, it follows that the metal flanges of these bridges will invariably stand away from the surfaces of the abutment teeth.

In the upper anterior region, these flanges may encroach on important guiding contacts and cause unwanted effects of occlusal interference. Here, the operator must establish the pattern of anterior guidance and decide whether or not to provide light contact on the flanges in intercuspal position and reproduce the guidance, or to create space and ignore anterior guidance entirely.

Indeed, it may not always be feasible or necessary to provide anterior guidance, because anterior teeth, restrained by the action of tongue, lip and intermittent 'functional' tooth contacts, need not drift or over-erupt. For practical reasons, the minimum thickness for strength of a non-perforated flange cast from a non-precious alloy is about 0.1–0.3 mm. It may be thicker for gold alloys and, unless there is a disclusion ('open bite') in the region, some tooth preparation may be necessary to prevent occlusal interferences occurring. Reduction of the tooth surfaces to accommodate anterior guidance should be planned carefully and not performed as an afterthought. Decision-making and occlusal planning are greatly simplified by mounting diagnostic casts on a semi-adjustable articulator.

For upper anterior bridges the following four situations should be considered.

No anterior guidance—open bite This poses no problems other than to ensure that the flanges are not too thick to encroach on the free space (Figures 5.17–5.19).

Short or shallow guidance (path less than 3.0 mm) It is probably best not to alter the occlusal relationship, but to let the margin of the flange bypass or circumvent the area of contact, provided, of course, this does not jeopardize the retentiveness of the flange itself (Figure 5.20).

Moderate guidance (path 3–5 mm) Either the enamel on the abutment teeth may be removed to accommodate the flange or, more simply, the opposing teeth may be reduced in height (Figure 5.21).

Long of steep guidance (path greater than 5.0 mm) This is the situation to avoid as far as possible because of the difficulties in accommodating the flanges without undue and excessive 'grinding' of the metal and the opposing teeth (Figures 5.22 and 5.23).

Careful planning is essential whenever reduction of the opposing teeth is intended. Preliminary assessment of guidance planes must be made with articulating tape. The thickness of enamel is not great—approximately 2.5 mm in the bulkier regions of the incisal edges and marginal ridges, and thinning out at the cervical area. Generally, the operator can expect to remove up to 1.0 mm thickness of enamel and still leave sufficient behind for etching. Practical details are given in Chapter 6.

Whether the 'inlay effect' has the same bearing on the bonding integrity of posterior bridges as it does on anterior bridges is open to speculation. It would not, however, be unreasonable to suppose that, given the greater extent of flange coverage that is possible in posterior teeth, the important occlusal contacts and guidance pathways (or guide paths) may be preserved without jeopardizing the bonds. For those patients with signs and symptoms of occlusal trauma, preliminary occlusal adjustment (equilibration) may be necessary and should be carried out competently before commencing bridgework. Occlusal therapy is outside the scope of this book and the interested reader should consult the many excellent textbooks published on the subject. Suffice it to say that the presence or absence of tooth contacts in posterior teeth, during protrusive and lateral excursions, should be determined before designing a posterior resin-bonded bridge.

Resistance and retention

Maximum resistance to lateral displacement forces is achieved by flange 'wrap-around' which may be described according to the angle subtended by the arc of the flange (Figure 5.24). For example, a wrap-around of 180 degrees would cover the entire lingual (or buccal) surface of the tooth from the mesial to the distal aspects (Figures 5.25–5.28).

Frequently, and particularly in posterior bridges, a buccal extension of metal (sometimes known as a 'buccal wrap') is provided giving a wrap-around of, for example, 225 degrees (Figure 5.29). Indeed, around conical teeth a full wrap of

[*contd on page 89*]

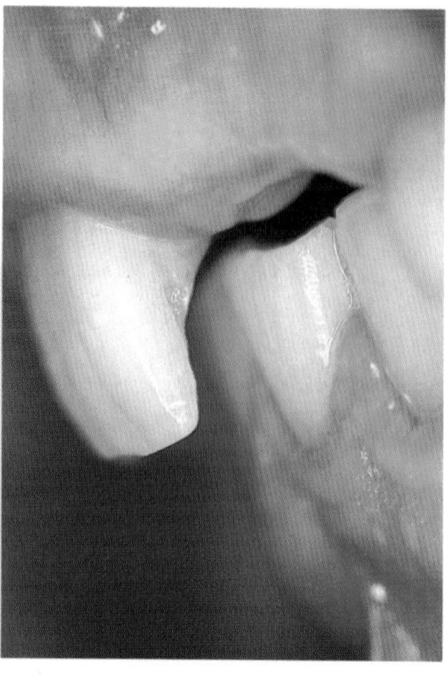
a

Figure 5.17

Absence of contact of lower incisors against the lingual aspects of upper incisors simplifies the design of resin-bonded bridges. (a, b) Incisal relationships in intercuspal position.

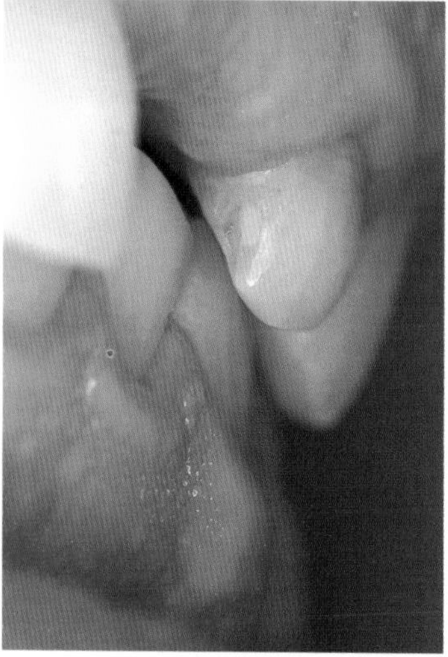
b

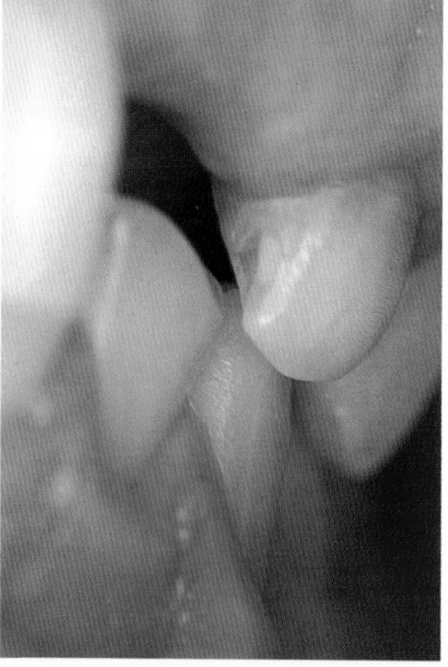
c

(c) Protrusive relationship of the upper left lateral incisor seen in (b) showing adequate clearance for a metal flange.

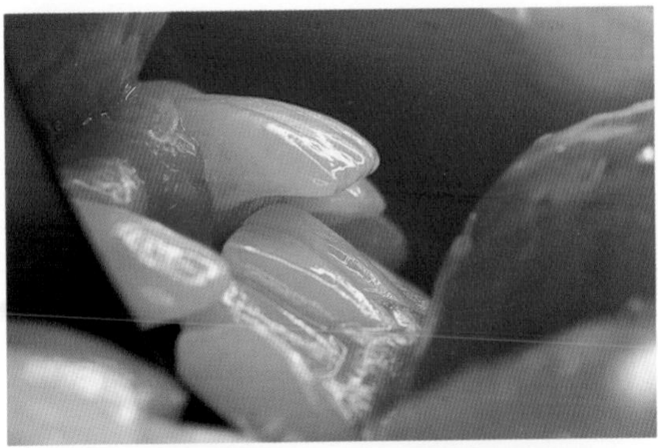
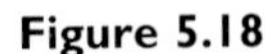

a

Figure 5.18

(a) In this patient there is sufficient clearance in intercuspal position and, although there is contact in anterior guidance on the incisal one-third (b), there would still be sufficient room for a metal flange.

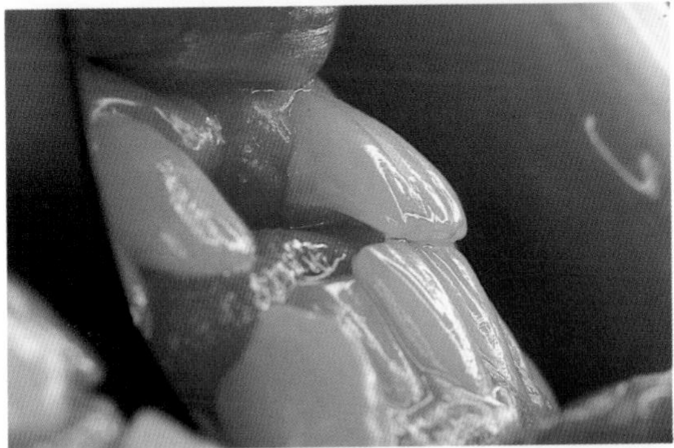

b

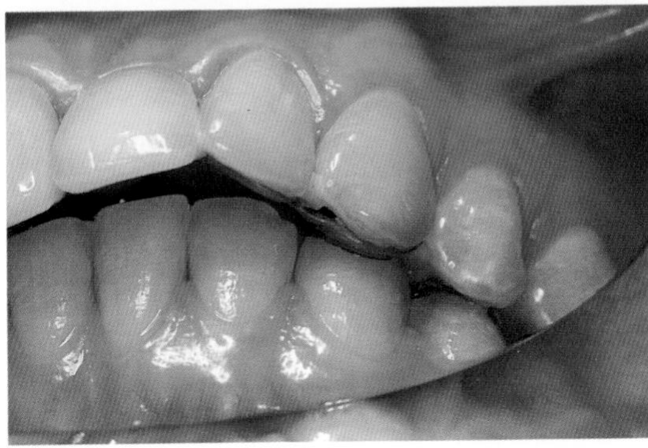

Figure 5.19

Thick flanges on the upper left lateral incisor and canine abutments have resulted in the obliteration of the free space and the introduction of interferences.

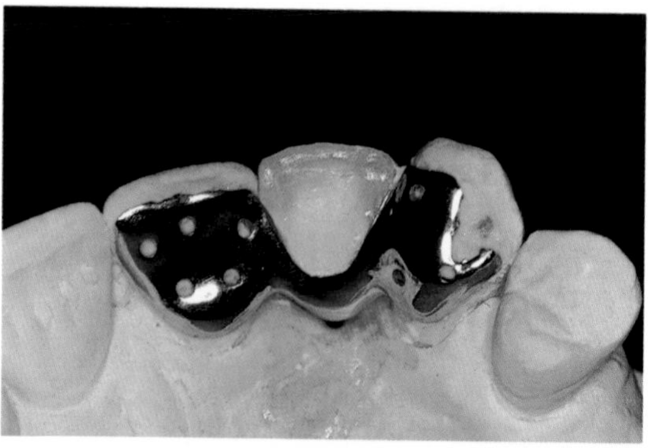

Figure 5.20

The flange on the upper left canine circumvents the occlusal guiding contact marked in blue.

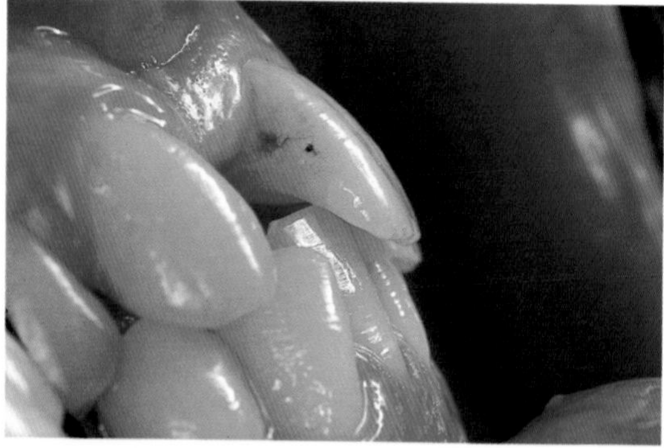

Figure 5.21

Moderate occlusal contact on upper incisors in intercuspal position.

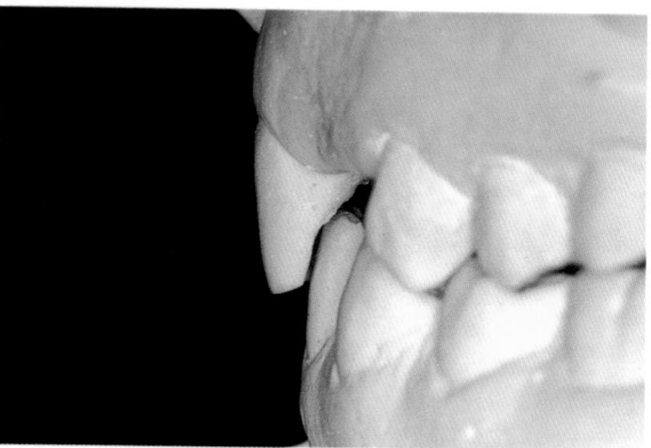

Figure 5.22

Steep guidance path on the upper incisors will increase difficulties of providing a resin-bonded bridge in this situation.

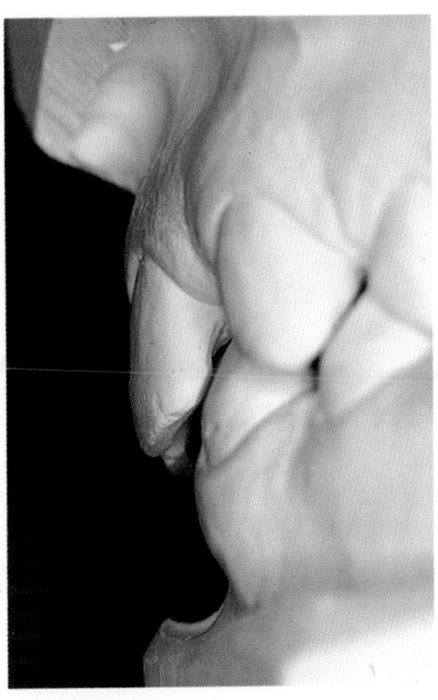

a

Figure 5.23

(a, b) A deep overbite in this young patient has reduced the space available for a metal flange.

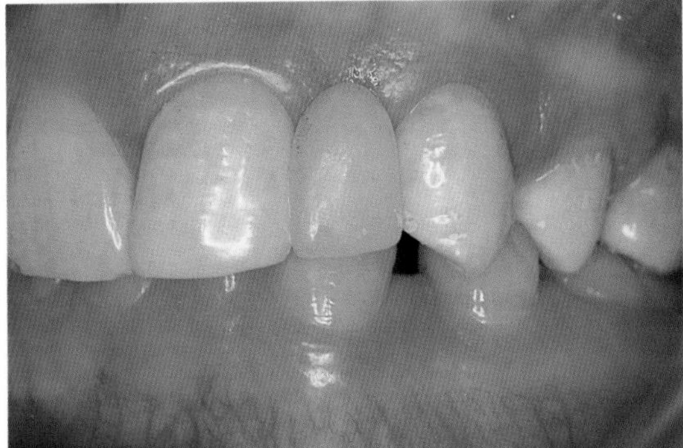

b

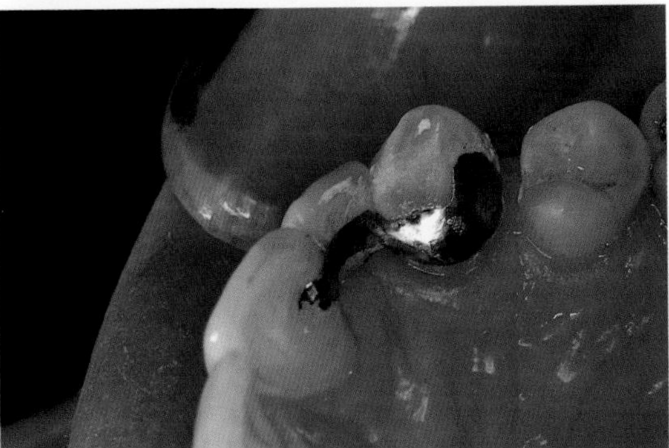

c

(c) This has resulted in the flange needing to be ground away due to lack of space.

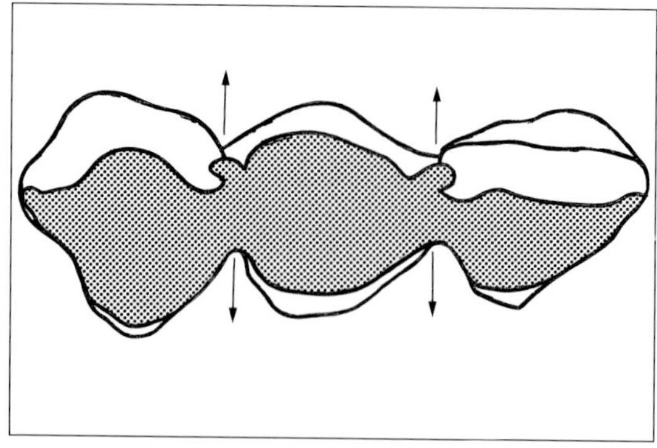

Figure 5.24

Diagram of suggested design of resin-bonded bridge with 180-degree 'wrap-around' and approximal grooves.

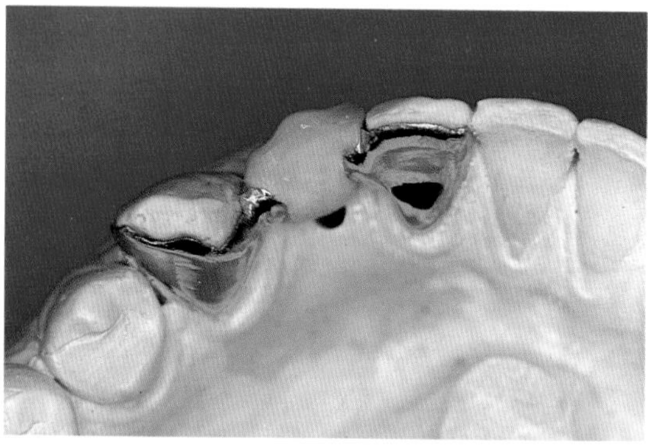

Figure 5.25

Wrap-around should be as extensive as aesthetic appearance would permit . . .

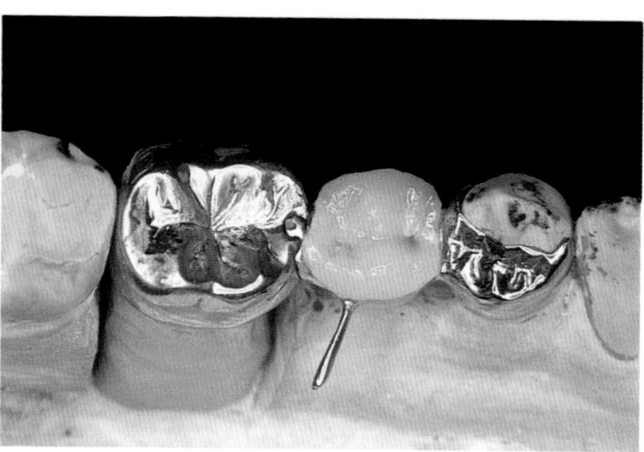

Figure 5.26

. . . even to the extent of covering cusps if the occlusion will allow, as in the lower first left premolar in this example. (Courtesy of Dr D.L. Hussey.)

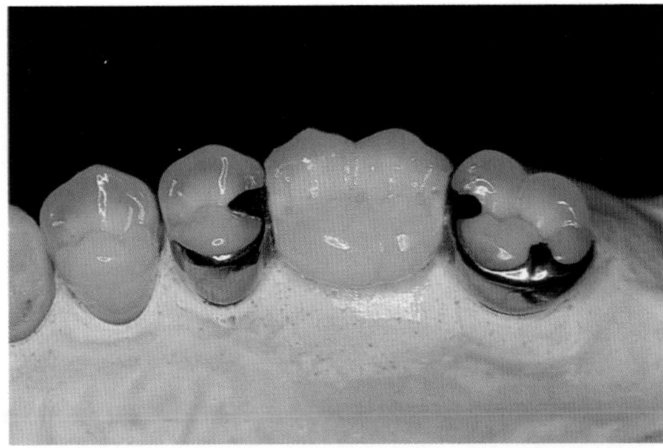

Figure 5.27

Occlusal rests provide good resistance and stability to displacing forces.

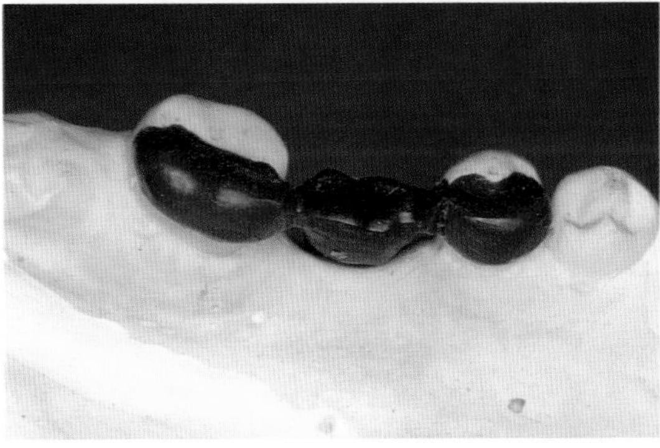

a

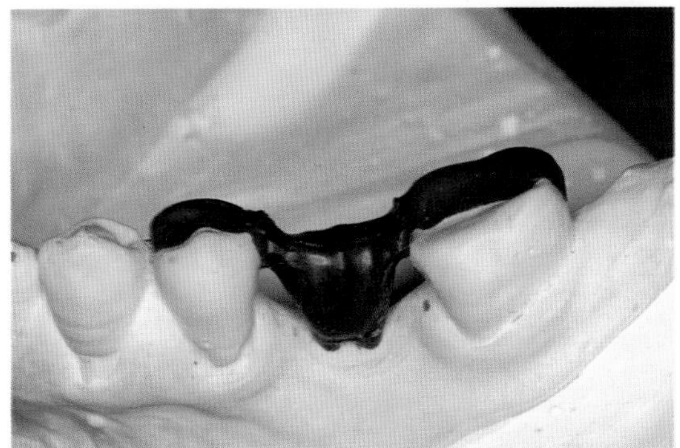

b

Figure 5.28 (a, b)

Wax-up of a fixed–fixed, resin-bonded bridge replacing lower left first molar. Note the coverage of the lingual cusps of the premolar and molar abutment teeth and good embrasure clearance in the pontic.

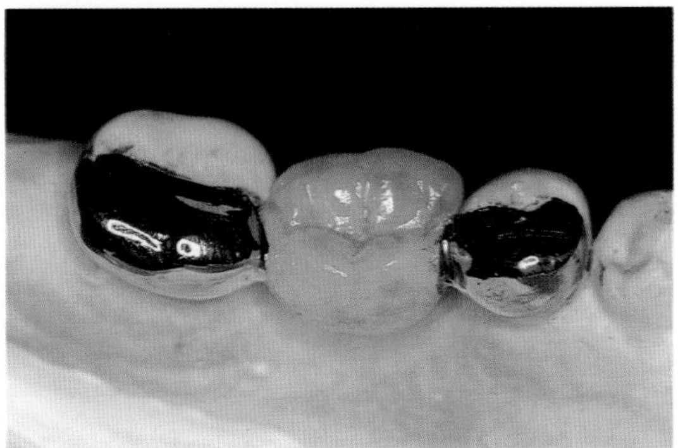

c

(c) The completed bridge. (Courtesy of Dr E. Lynch.)

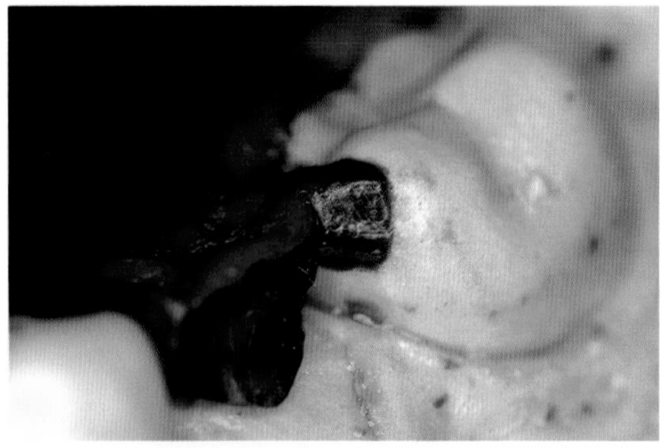

Figure 5.29

Where appropriate in posterior teeth, buccal extensions may enhance retention and stability.

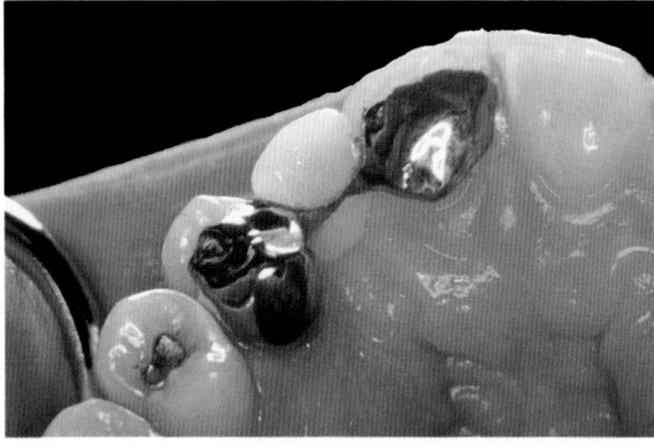

Figure 5.30

In this patient, almost total occlusal coverage was possible on the upper right first premolar owing to the absence of occlusal contacts with the opposing tooth.

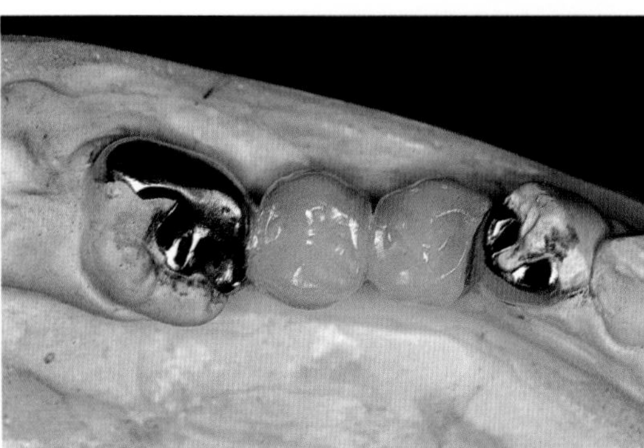

Figure 5.31

Owing to an excessive lingual inclination of the lower left second molar, a buccal 'wrap' was created instead.

360 degrees is possible. Where there is no interference from the occlusion, it is advantageous to cover the lingual cusps of posterior abutment teeth (Figure 5.30 and see Figures 5.25 and 5.27). Obviously, natural tooth undercuts may impede the insertion of the bridge and it may be necessary to shift the 'wrap' to another surface (Figure 5.31). It is always advisable to survey the diagnostic casts in order to determine the optimum path of insertion and enable planned reduction of the tooth surfaces (Figure 5.32).

Wrap-around extensions are obviously constrained by the aesthetic requirement in the anterior region. A bizarre example of an overzealous adherence to the wrap-around principle is illustrated in Figure 5.33. Nevertheless, where it is feasible 'wraps' would provide good resistance to displacement and a determinate path of insertion for the bridge, and would enhance the flexural resistance of the framework.

The provision of occlusal rests in posterior teeth, cingulum ledges in anterior teeth and approximal grooves in either offers good retention and resistance. Similarly, where the flange extends onto the marginal ridge or over a cusp, a firm resistance to gingival displacement is provided (see Figures 5.27 and 5.30).

Whether or not the teeth should be cut to provide these features is, however, a contentious issue. Proponents maintain that tooth preparation or modification ensures a distinct path of insertion which enhances location and retention. In this, they are supported by mounting clinical evidence that the success rate is increased where prior tooth preparation had been carried out (Barrack, 1984; Eshleman et al, 1984; Clyde and Boyd, 1988; Burgess and McCartney, 1989). Opponents argue that tooth preparation is unnecessary and negates the *raison d'être* of resin-bonded bridges which is to dispel the fear of 'drilling' and fulfil its designation as a 'non-preparation' bridge. At any rate, the intention, as far as possible, is to confine the preparation within the enamel and not to expose dentine.

Tooth preparation

A good example of the need for tooth preparation, to assist in the correct location of the bridge, may be seen in the lower incisor region where the teeth tend to be tall, slim and with steep lingual slopes, and are likely to present indeterminate paths of insertion for a bridge (Figure 5.34). When cementing such a bridge, the lubricating effect of the luting resin makes it difficult to ascertain the correct seating of the bridge by touch. Only after excess set cement has been removed will the disconcerting discovery of a 'misfit' be made (Figure 5.35).

Design for tooth preparations

The design of tooth preparations may be considered under the following headings:

1 Circumferential reduction.
2 Palatal/occlusal reduction.
3 Finish lines.
4 Vertical rests or stops.
5 Vertical grooves and/or pins.

Circumferential reduction

Part of the general design of the wrap-around feature is the reduction of the surfaces of the abutment teeth. After a survey of the study casts to determine the maximum contours of the abutment teeth, reduction is carried out with tapered or torpedo-shaped diamond stones (Figure 5.36). A two-plane reduction, with extensions on the labial/buccal and palatal/lingual aspects, is generally favoured (Figures 5.37 and 5.38). This effectively removes approximately 0.5–1 mm of surface enamel. Obviously, in the anterior teeth the reduction has to be fairly judicious for aesthetic reasons, but no such constraints exist in the preparation of posterior teeth, where the 'wrap' may be as extensive as required by the need for maximum resistance to displacement forces (Figure 5.39).

Palatal/occlusal reduction

The reduction of palatal and occlusal surfaces is carried out to accommodate occlusal contacts and guide planes, and has been considered in detail under *occlusal contacts*.

Finish lines

Some operators prefer a light but distinct chamfer to delineate the margins of the flange (see Figures

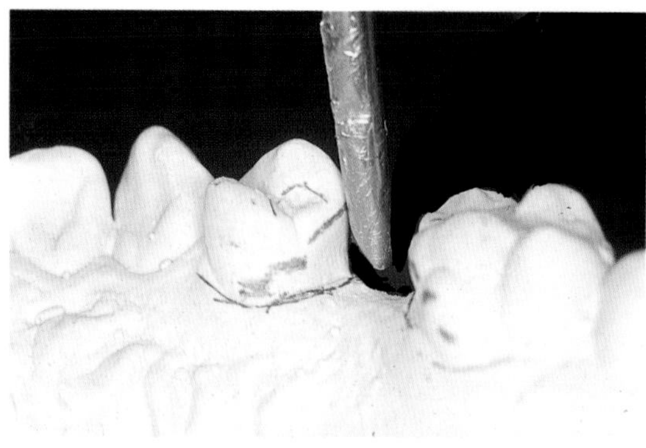

Figure 5.32

It is good practice to survey study casts before designing a resin-bonded bridge.

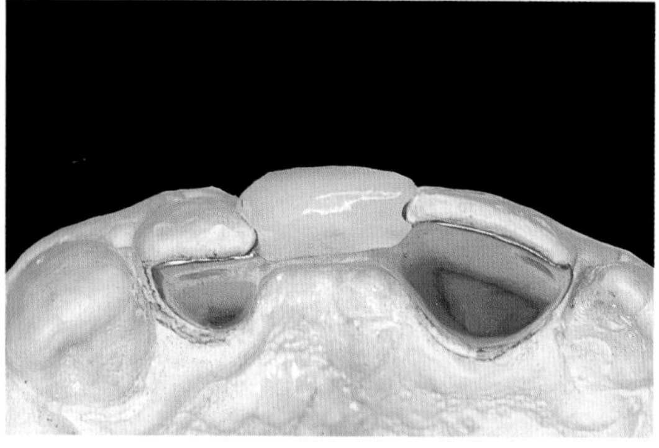

a

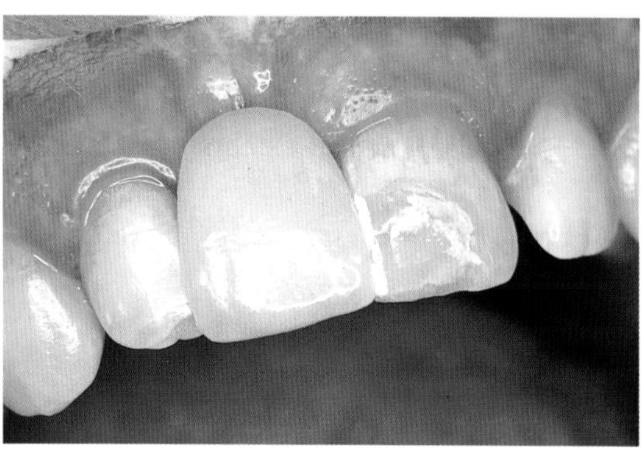

b

Figure 5.33 (a, b)

Overzealous wrap-around in this bridge has created a grotesque appearance of the upper right incisor pontic.

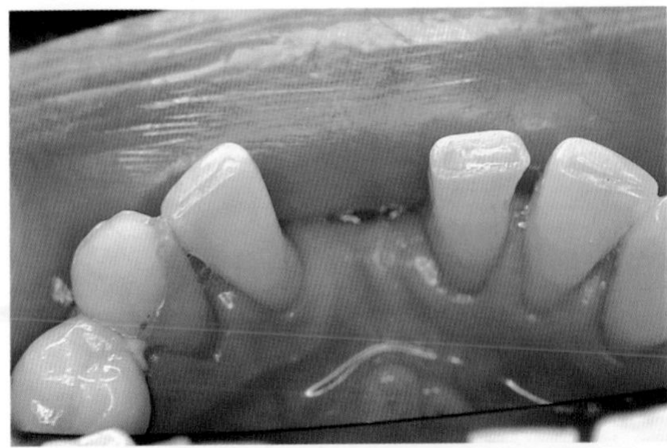

Figure 5.34

The lower incisor, being tall and slender, may not provide determinate paths of insertion for a bridge.

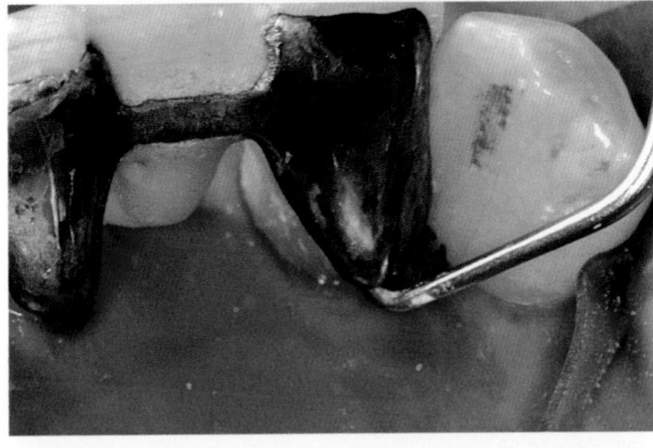

Figure 5.35

Here, misalignment of a lower anterior resin-bonded bridge was only discovered after cementation.

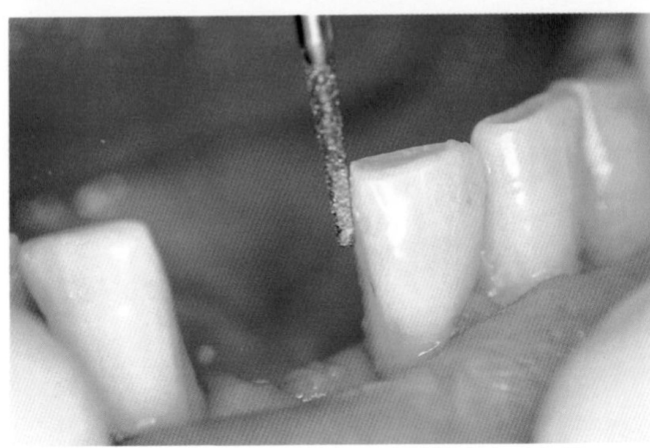

Figure 5.36

Approximal groove preparation with a long tapered diamond bur.

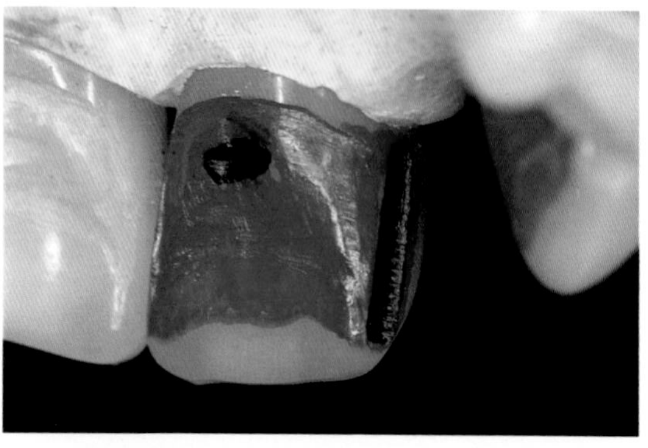

a

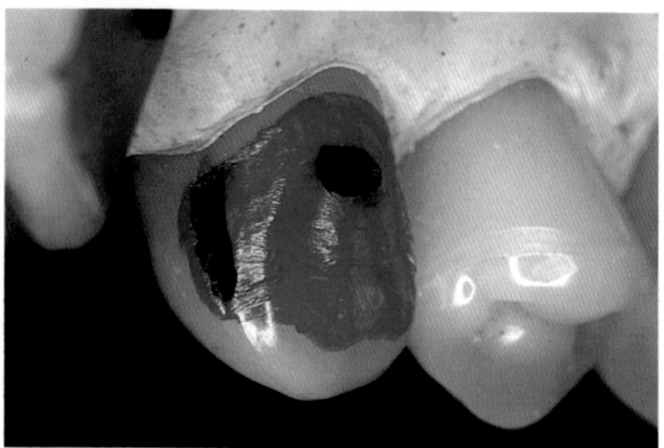

b

Figure 5.37 (a, b)

Tooth preparation illustrating cingulum rests, approximal grooves and fine chamfer margins.

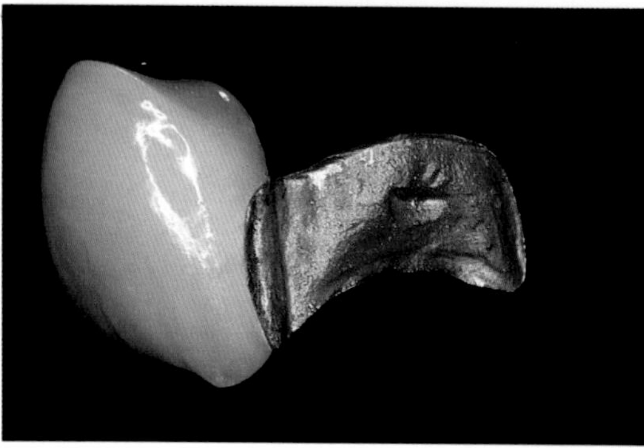

Figure 5.38

Casting showing detail of grooves, cingulum rest and chamfer margin.

5.37 and 5.38). The finish lines are always placed supragingivally and create a definite limit to which the technician may wax the flange pattern. In addition, it is possible that superficial, aprismatic enamel which is difficult to etch may be removed during the preparation of the chamfer. Consequently, the underlying prismatic and highly etchable enamel is exposed, thus ensuring a secure bond to the luting resin (Aker et al, 1979).

Vertical rests or stops

Vertical rest seats may be placed on a marginal ridge, occlusal fossa or cusp (see Figures 5.26–5.31) and, in the anterior teeth, on the cingulum (Figures 5.37, 5.38 and 5.40). Cingulum rests are usually notch-shaped and placed over the bulkiest part of the cingulum. The number, size and position of occlusal rests depend on how much stability is already achieved by wrap-around, and of course by occlusal contacts of the opposing teeth. If the lingual cusps can be covered, then obviously there is no need for additional rests. The cusp of Carabelli in the upper first molars is particularly suitable as an occlusal rest. As a general rule, at least one rest per tooth should be placed and this should be cut to a depth of approximately 1.0–1.5 mm (depending on the available thickness of enamel) with distinct walls to resist lateral movement (Figures 5.41 and 5.42).

Vertical grooves and pins

The function of vertical grooves or channels is similar to that in partial veneer-cast metal crowns, ie to resist rotational or 'torquing' forces. Grooves are usually placed in pairs and act reciprocally. To be effective, they must be parallel to one another, have definite lingual walls and must be contained within the margins of the casting (see Figures 5.37 and 5.38). The grooves adjacent to the pontic may be placed as far labially or buccally as the 'wrap' margin will permit. Also, the longer the grooves, the more retentive they will be within the same constraint.

In resin-bonded bridges, the construction of grooves is generally only possible on the surface adjacent to the saddle area because of the limitation of the contact surfaces distal to the saddle. Nevertheless, sufficient height may be gained if the 'distal' groove is placed in the vicinity of a cusp or cingulum (Figure 5.43). A recommendation by Yamashita and Yamani (1986) is to position these reciprocal grooves at opposite ends of an imaginary line drawn across the bonding surface, whose midpoint lies over the long axis of the tooth (Figure 5.44). Needless to say, these grooves should be cut only in enamel, although exposure of some dentine is not disastrous. As such, the grooves tend to be broader than those of conventional partial veneer crowns, and may be cut with a suitable tungsten carbide or diamond bur.

In difficult situations where the amount of bonding surface may be reduced, such as in partially erupted teeth, or where persistent detachment ('debonding') has occurred for whatever reason, the use of pins to enhance retention may be adopted (Wiltshire, 1986b; Lynn, 1987). Obviously, this has to be carried out most carefully, and a prior knowledge of pulp form and position which may be gleaned from radiographs is essential. The depth and location of pin channels are limited in scope. Generally, 2 mm depth is the maximum that should be attempted without penetrating too deeply into dentine. In the maxillary anterior teeth, pins can be placed safely just mesial or distal to the cingulum, and in upper and lower premolars and molars, alongside the mesial or distal marginal ridges at a position usually occupied by an occlusal rest. Of course, the pin may be an integral part of the occlusal rest itself.

Pins may be part of the casting, in which case they must have the same path of insertion as the rest of the retainer, or they may be placed along different lines of insertion after cementation of the bridge, thereby 'locking' the retainers in position. To some operators this may seem the more logical approach, because the retention available would be far greater than that afforded by parallel grooves, and would only be limited by the shear strength of the pins or screws used. However, one disadvantage is that, should a failure in the resin-to-metal or resin-to-enamel bond occur, it may be difficult to remove the bridge for reclamation or renovation. In the main, auxiliary pin retention should be reserved for persistent bonding failures.

Existing restorations

In anterior teeth, the presence of small approximal or lingual composite resin restorations does

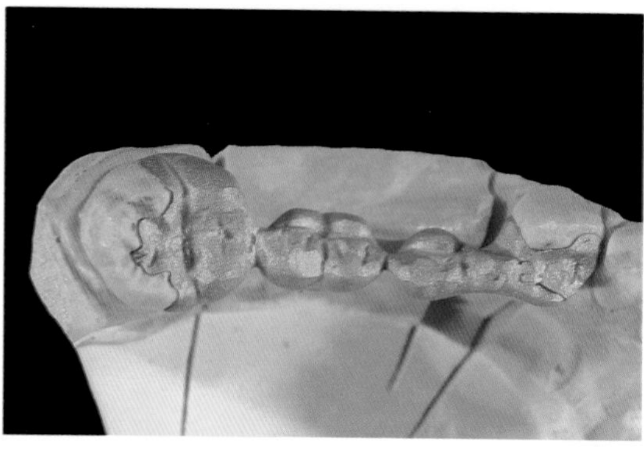

Figure 5.39

Extensive coverage of retainers is essential for maximum stability in long-span bridges. (Courtesy of Dr A.C. Shortall.)

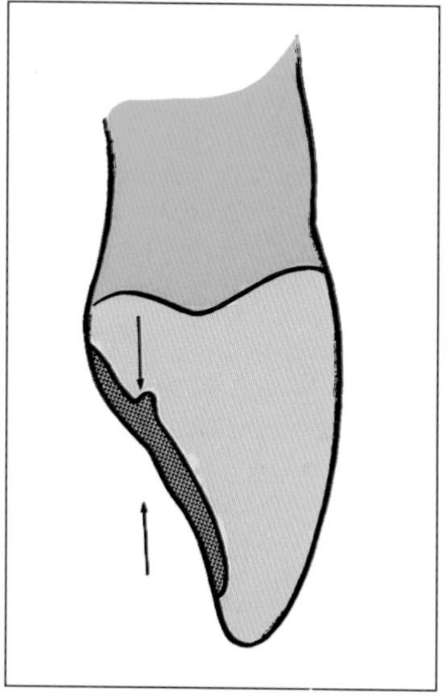

Figure 5.40

Diagram showing the effect of cingulum rest seats in upper anterior teeth in resisting vertical displacing forces.

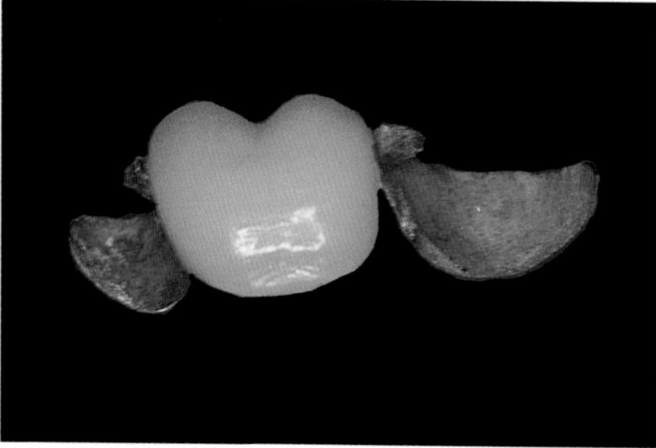

Figure 5.41

Occlusal rests should have distinct walls provided by rest seats cut in the tooth to resist displacement.

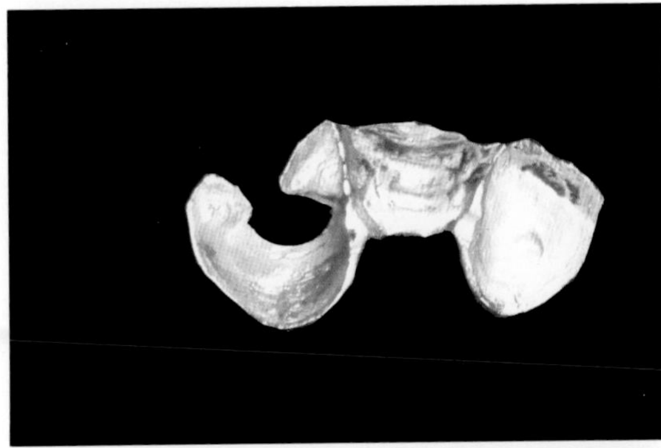

Figure 5.42

Casting of a resin-bonded bridge showing occlusal rests with sufficient bulk.

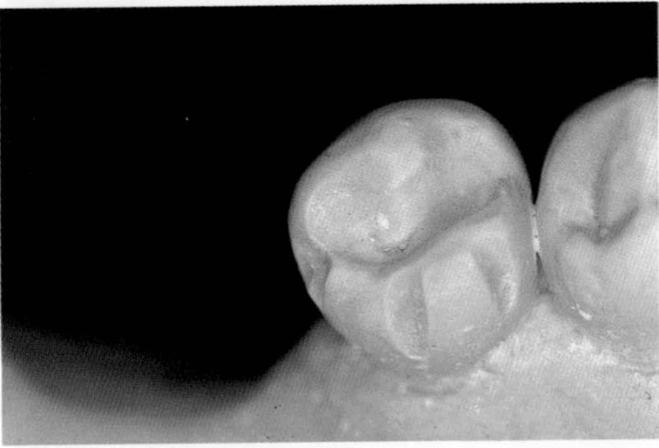

a

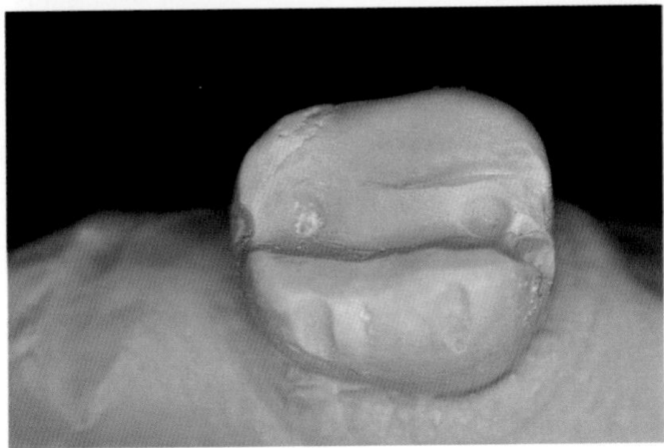

b

Figure 5.43 (a, b)

Maximum height of grooves is achieved if they are placed within the vicinity of cusps.

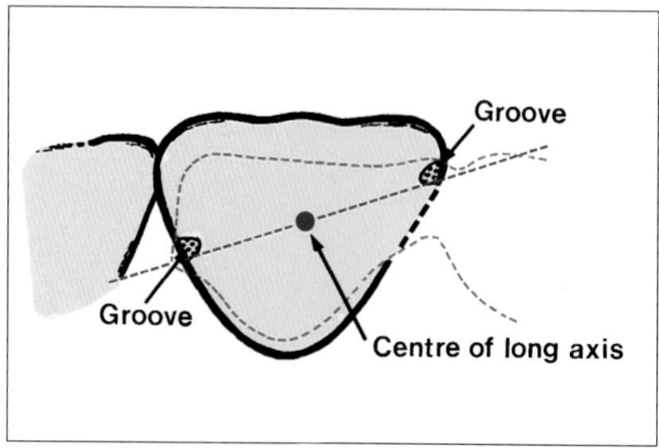

a

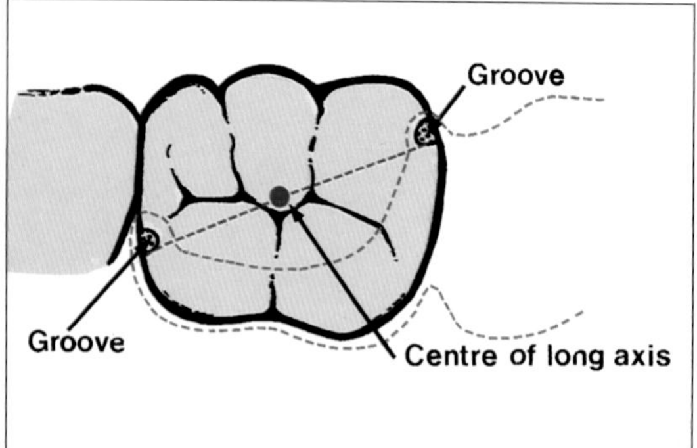

b

Figure 5.44 (a, b)

Diagrams showing position of reciprocating grooves, as suggested by Yamashita and Yamani (1986).

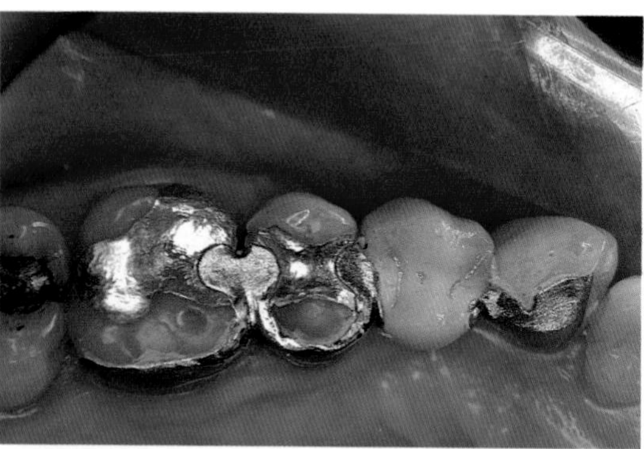

Figure 5.45

Due to the lack of adhesion between resin and amalgam, occlusal rests should be placed well within the boundaries of the amalgam restoration.

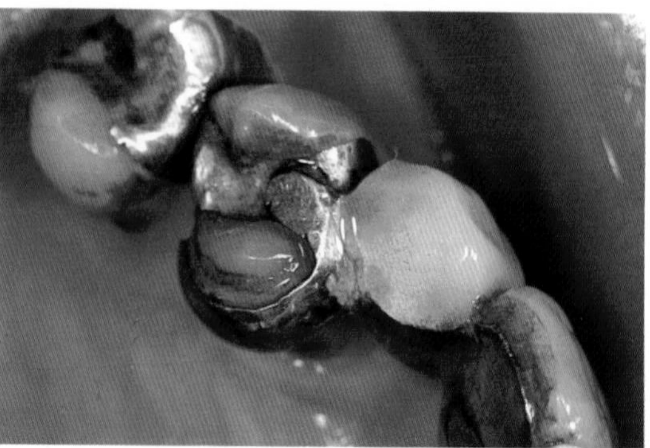

Figure 5.46

The occlusal rest in this bridge was placed too close to the amalgam margin. This imposes a risk of caries developing due to the potential stagnation area.

not have to be detrimental to the bridge. Ideally, the margins of the flange should extend beyond the margins of the restoration to avoid the complications of microleakage. If the restoration is defective, it should be replaced with a new composite resin or glass-ionomer restoration. Before cementing the bridge in place, the surface of the restoration should be roughened slightly, and cleaned and etched along with the rest of the enamel of the tooth.

Small occlusal amalgam restorations in posterior teeth may be bypassed if they do not encroach on the marginal ridges or areas where occlusal rests are planned. In premolars, occlusal pit amalgam restorations may even be removed and the existing cavity used to enhance resistance and retention after it is first lined with a calcium hydroxide base or a glass-ionomer lining cement. Both these lining materials are now available in the light-curing form, which have been shown in laboratory tests to be more durable and easier to handle than their autosetting counterparts.

Whilst it may be possible to place occlusal rests on existing amalgam restorations (Figures 5.45 and 5.46), in general it would be inadvisable due to the lack of bond between resin and metal which gives rise to microleakage that may in turn lead to caries; this is particularly the case if the margins of the rests were in close proximity to the margins of the amalgam restoration. Eventually, debonding of the retainers may occur. The introduction of special primers which purport to enhance the bond between resin and amalgam may prove to be beneficial, but as yet little evidence is available.

Large, poorly contoured or leaky amalgam restorations in abutment teeth should be replaced, preferably with one of the new 'posterior composite resins', which are usually of the 'hybrid' or 'macrofilled' types. Figure 5.47 illustrates a case where an existing, large, pin-retained, amalgam restoration has been partially removed and replaced with a composite resin to provide an 'attractive' bonding surface for the metal flange.

If the existing restoration is satisfactory, it need not be removed, but the occlusal rests or margins of the retainer should avoid the restoration margins to prevent microleakage. Where this is not feasible, then a small 'inlay box' may be cut in the restoration, extending to the enamel walls which, when etched, may furnish bonds to the composite resin lute (Figure 5.48).

The presence of existing crowns on potential abutment teeth presents added complications. Assuming that the occlusal relationships are favourable, several options may be considered.

Where both the mesial and distal abutments are to be crowned

In the situation it may, on balance, be advisable not to consider a resin-bonded bridge, but to design a conventional one.

Where a crown is planned for either of the abutment teeth

Either a 'hybrid' bridge with a movable joint in the crowned tooth or a cantilevered design may be adopted. In the hybrid design (Figure 5.49), it is important that the female part (matrix) of the attachment is located in the crown. Should debonding accidentally occur, it would be a simple matter to remove the resin-bonded part for servicing and rebonding.

Where a lateral incisor is to be replaced and the canine abutment is sound, a cantilever bridge off the canine is the treatment of choice when the central incisor abutment has an existing crown. It is not a good idea to cut a slot in the distal aspect of the crown to create a movable joint, because the fact that the slot must be cut deeply enough to provide good resistance to displacement forces creates problems. There is a danger that accidental perforation of the crown may occur where its internal dimensions are unknown. Equally, the central incisor may be used as an abutment to cantilever a lateral incisor pontic if the canine is unusable.

A central incisor pontic may be cantilevered from its fellow incisor when the lateral incisor is otherwise crowned. It may also be feasible to design a spring cantilever bridge from the sound canine with the central incisor pontic carried on a palatal bar which bypasses the crowned lateral incisor completely.

In the posterior arch, where aesthetic considerations are less complicated, it may be possible to modify the crowned abutment to accept a 360-degree wrap-around. As mentioned in Chapter 2, it would be feasible to construct a porcelain veneer bridge to mate with the existing porcelain crowns of the abutment teeth (see Figure 2.45).

Root-filled teeth as prospective abutments

There is no contraindication to the use of root-filled teeth as abutments, provided the root filling is well condensed, the apical seal intact and there is no evidence of apical abnormalities. In fact, extra retention may be gained by extending the flange into the access cavity as a short post (Figure 5.50). The main problem would appear to be the discoloration of the labial surface of the tooth which is often a feature of non-vital teeth. This may be treated with initial peroxide bleaching of the crown followed by placement of a porcelain or composite resin veneer (Figure 5.50a,c). If discoloration sets in after the bridge has been fitted, it may still be masked with a veneer without removal of the bridge, provided the discoloration is not too severe (Figure 5.51).

Physiological form

The physiological form of the bridge is related to the maintenance of a stable occlusion and the preservation of gingival and periodontal health. The effect of occlusion has been mentioned; here, the influence of the topography of the retainer flange on the health of the periodontal tissues will be discussed under the headings: location and quality of the margins, and surface contour of the flange.

Location and quality of the margins The location of the margins in relation to the gingival tissues is a major factor in the maintenance of periodontal health. There is ample clinical evidence to show that margins placed supragingivally cause less inflammation of the gingivae than subgingival margins. Even with well-fitting margins, if these were placed subgingivally, greater gingival reaction could be expected, sometimes leading to loss of epithelial attachment and deepening of the sulcus. Plaque accumulation around both sub- and supragingival margins is probably the same; the difference occurs in the degree of gingival inflammation caused. As a general rule, the margin of a resin-bonded bridge flange should be placed about 1mm away from the gingival margin.

Rough, ill-fitting margins alone may not damage the periodontium as such, but do so indirectly by increasing the chances of plaque accumulation and thereby gingival inflammation.

A smooth, knife-edge margin, resting intimately on the enamel surface and interposed by a thin resin lute (that is, <15 μm thick), would appear to be satisfactory. Whether or not this ideal can be achieved clinically is doubtful. Several operators have suggested that a minimal chamfer preparation, approximately 0.1 mm deep around the cervical margin, may assist both in the achievement of closeness of fit and in the prevention of overcontouring (Simonsen et al, 1983).

Surface contour of the flange In conventional crowns and bridges, a proper contour of the retainers is generally regarded as essential for good periodontal health. However, as yet there is no consensus in the literature as to what constitutes the ideal crown contour that is best tolerated by the gingival tissues.

Some authorities believe that a slight cervical bulge would deflect the bolus of food during mastication to 'massage' the soft tissues instead of the bolus being driven directly into the gingival sulcus, perhaps causing stagnation. Unfortunately, this combined stimulating and self-cleansing concept has virtually no scientific evidence to support it (Pameijer, 1985).

However, others have claimed that a pronounced cervical contour encourages plaque accumulation and actually hinders cleansing. Indeed, rather than protect the gingivae, cervical overcontour may protect the bacterial plaque instead.

Unless gross enamel reduction is carried out to accommodate the thickness of the casting, the lingual flange of a resin-bonded bridge would be overcontoured anyway. It has not been firmly established whether or not this has any significant bearing on plaque retention, although a recent short-term clinical survey indicated that plaque accumulation around overcontoured flanges was not markedly increased, provided the flange margins were placed at least 1mm above the gingival crest (Creugers et al, 1988). On the whole, undercontouring is preferable because there is considerable clinical evidence to suggest that such a surface would reduce plaque accumulation and facilitate plaque removal.

Using movable joints

The incorporation of a movable joint within the bridge would, at first sight, impugn the requirement

[*contd on page 105*]

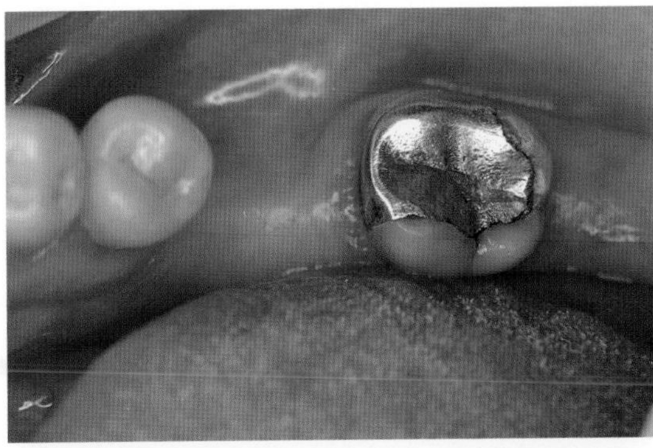

Figure 5.47

Replacement of part of a pin-retained amalgam restoration in the lower right second molar with a hybrid composite resin (Herculite, Kerr) to accommodate a resin-bonded bridge flange. (a) Preoperative state;

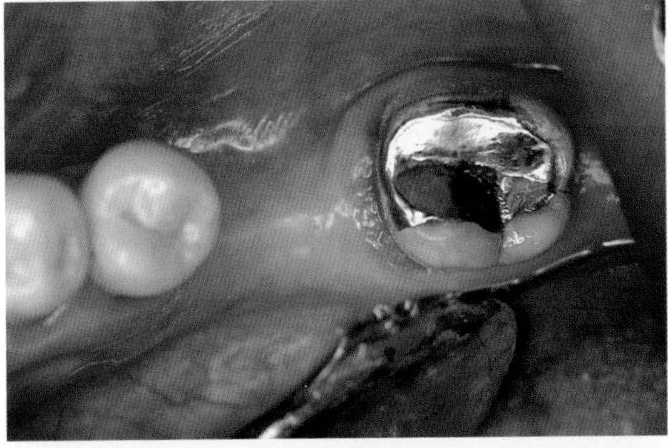

(b) amalgam polished;

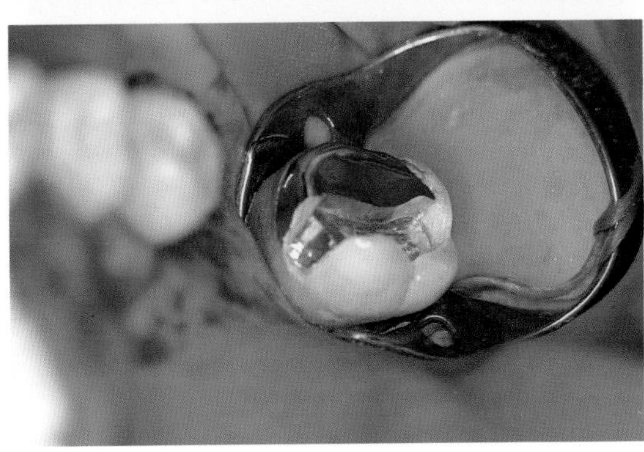

(c) cavity prepared to receive composite resin;

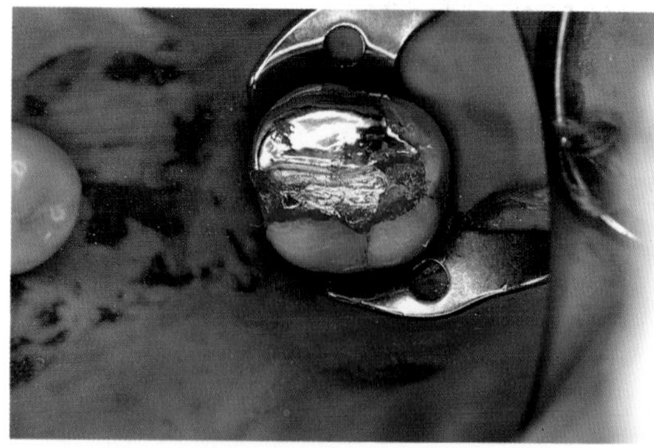

(d) margins etched;

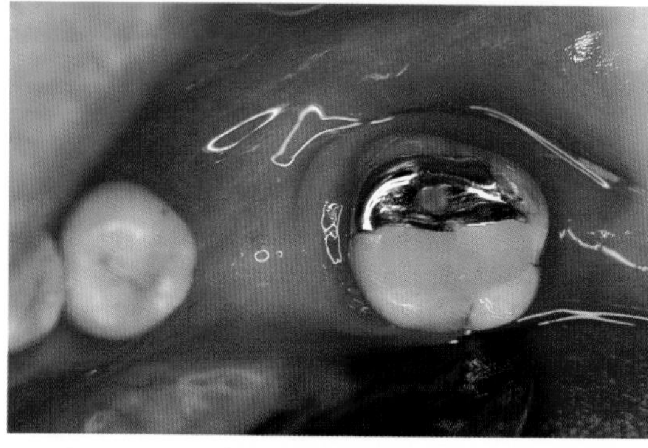

(e) composite placed and finished;

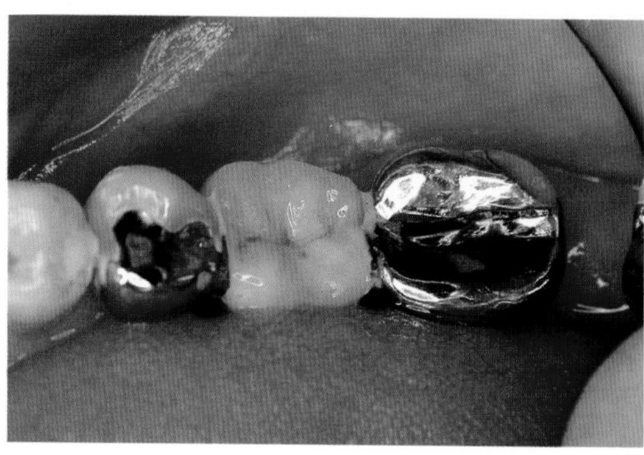

(f) completed fixed–movable bridge in place. (Courtesy of Dr E. Lynch.)

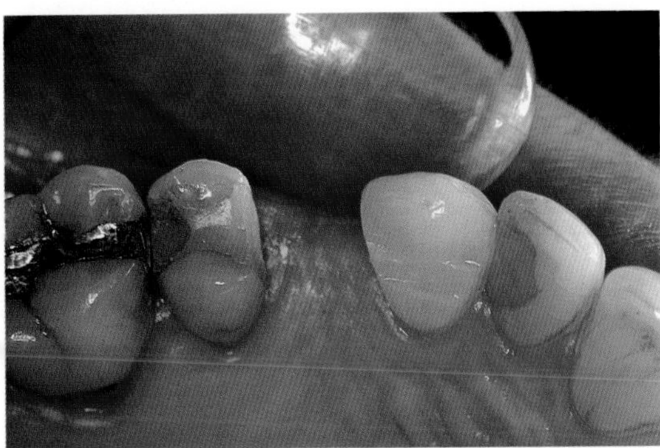

Figure 5.48

(a) Small inlay box cut within composite resin restoration in upper right second premolar to accommodate occlusal rest of the bridge.

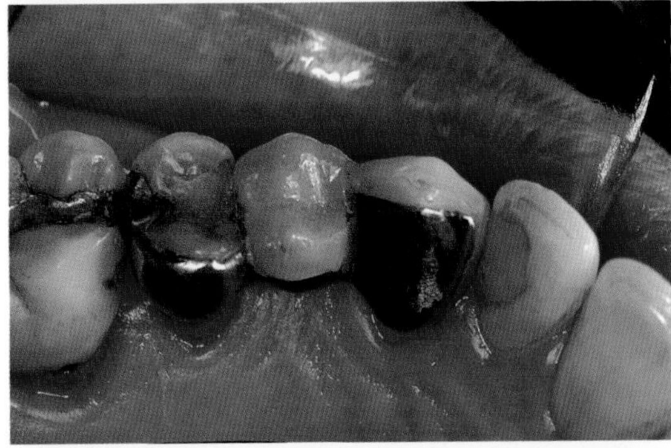

(b) The enamel margins of the box are exposed to be etched so as to provide a good bond to the resin cement.

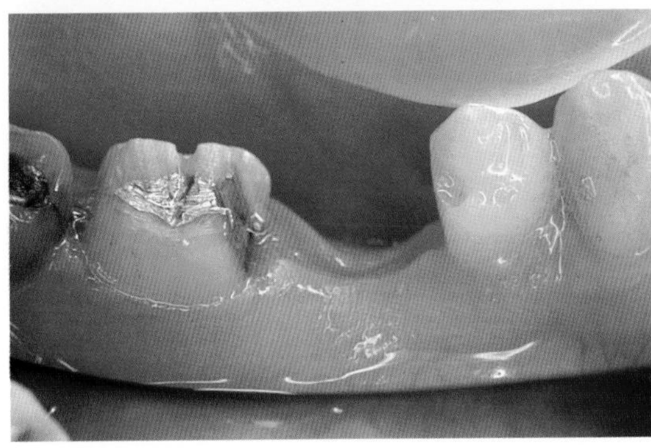

Figure 5.49

(a) Crown preparation for a hybrid resin-bonded bridge.

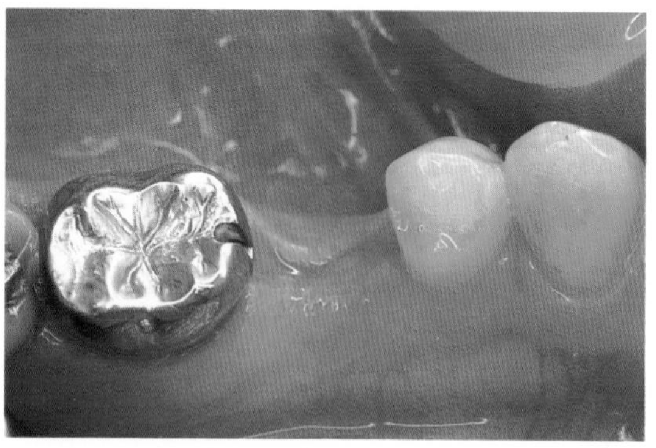

(b) The 'female' component (matrix) of the non-rigid attachment should be incorporated in the conventional crown.

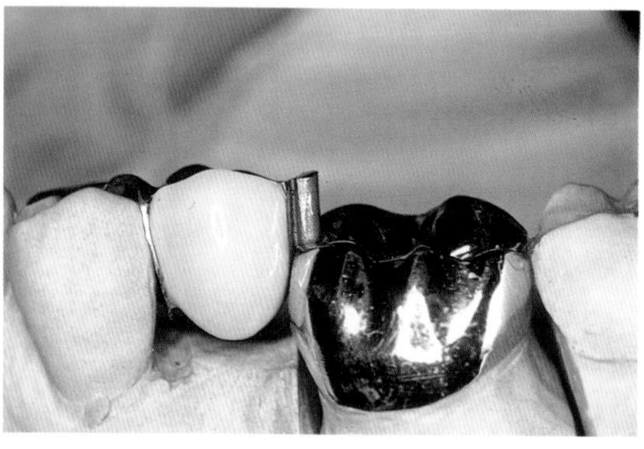

(c) Buccal view showing 'male' component (patrix) sliding into the matrix.

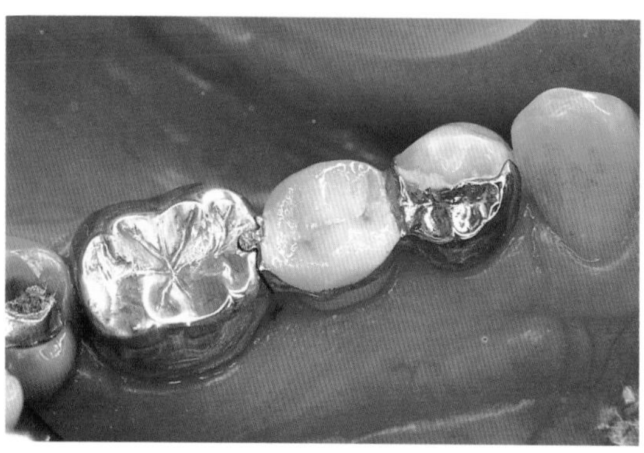

(d) Completed bridge in place. (Courtesy of Dr D.L. Hussey.)

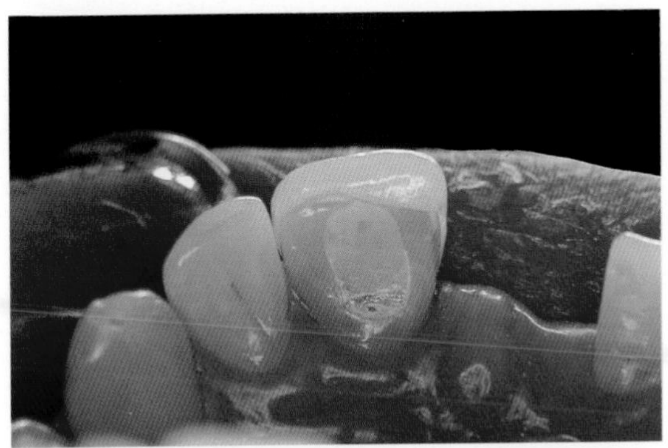

a

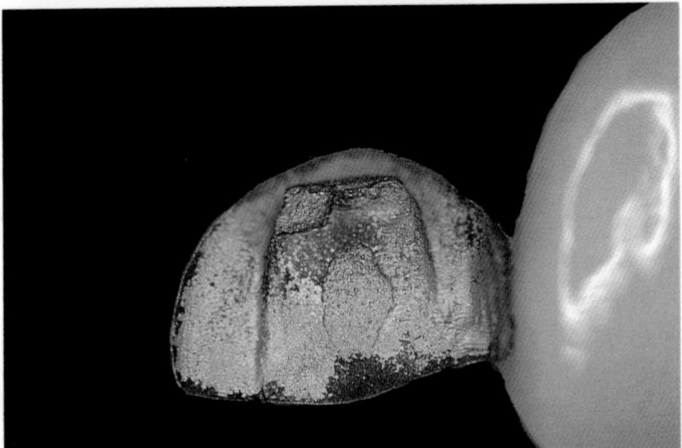

b

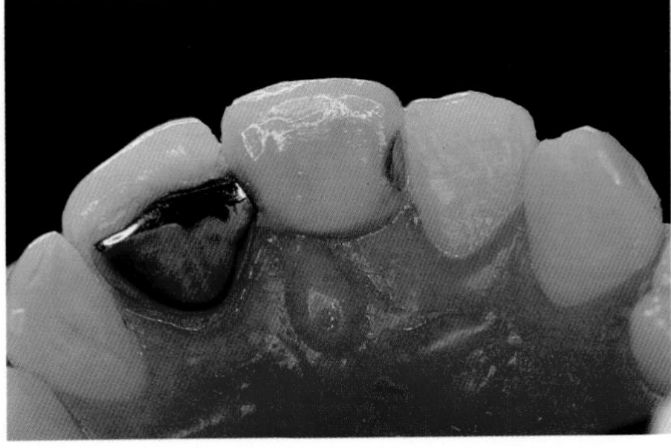

c

Figure 5.50

(a) Root-filled, upper right central incisor with lingual cavity prepared to receive a short post-extension of the flange (b). This proved to be sufficiently retentive for this bridge to be converted into a cantilever design when the flange on the upper left lateral incisor had debonded (c) (see also Figure 6.25a).

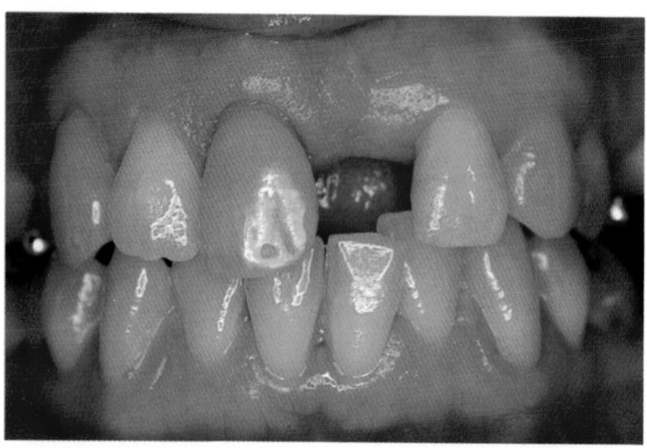

Figure 5.51

Discoloration of upper right central incisor abutment corrected with a porcelain veneer. (a) Preoperative state;

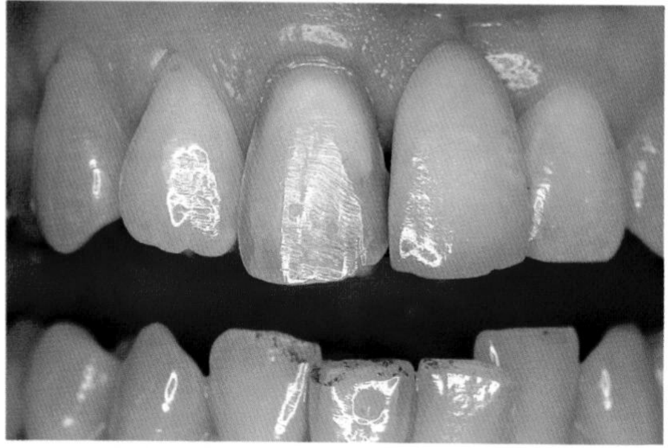

(b) veneer preparation after bridge had been fitted;

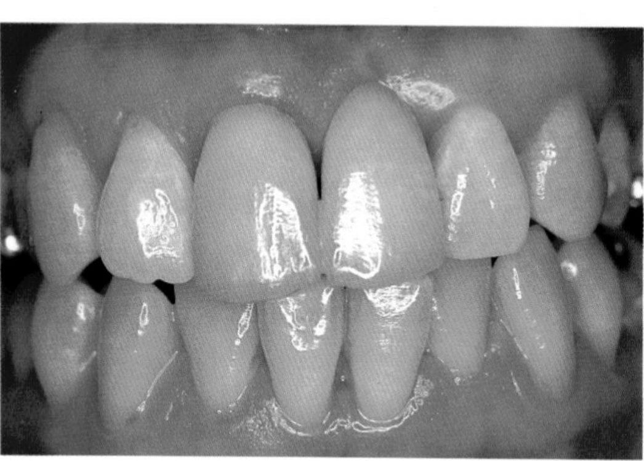

(c) veneer in place.

of a rigid framework. However, in conventional bridgework it is known that where there are retainers with differing retentive capacities, the one with the least retention is the one most likely to fail and become loose. To counteract this, a movable joint is incorporated in the framework to effect a 'stress-breaking' action between the two parts of the bridge. This applies to resin-bonded bridges, particularly where the abutment teeth display differing degrees of mobility, eg across a cleft palate (Figure 5.52). To counteract this, a movable joint is incorporated to effect a 'stress-breaking' action between the two parts of the bridge. Owing to lack of space in the retainers, these attachments are sometimes placed within the pontic, ideally approaching on the lingual aspect to maintain proper embrasure spaces (Figure 5.52c,d).

In addition, the longer the span of the bridge, the greater its flexion. With bridges with a long span, it may be difficult to obtain a single path of insertion due to natural tooth undercuts. Removal of these undercuts by tooth preparation may be hazardous and jeopardize the etch technique. It seems appropriate that, in these situations, splitting the bridge into two segments via a movable attachment will impart a degree of independent movement on the segments thereby reducing the chances of failure (Figures 5.53 and 5.54).

Pontic design

The design of the pontic is often said to be a compromise between its ability to be cleansed and appearance. Which way the bias shifts depends on the part of the mouth in which the bridge is placed, but generally it is 'cleansability' that should hold sway.

Two favoured designs are the dome-shaped (*synonyms*: bullet-shaped, torpedo-shaped) pontic and the modified ridge lap pontic. The former is so called because its gingival aspect is smooth and rounded with minimum mucosal contact at the crest of the ridge (Figure 5.55). Wide embrasures are possible approximally, and patients have no difficulty in cleaning this bridge. With skill, a trained technician may produce very acceptable results even in the anterior region, but on the whole, dome-shaped pontics are usually confined to the posterior region of the mouth.

The modified ridge lap pontic is a compromise between appearance and cleansability, and there is minimal soft tissue contact on the labial or buccal aspect of the ridge (Figures 5.56 and 5.57).

A full saddle pontic, so named because it sits astride the ridge and has by far the greatest area of tissue contact, is the least favoured design within some authorities due to the inflammation it can cause, especially if the now-discredited practice of scraping off the mucosal contact area on the stone cast is carried out. However, others feel that, because plaque can cause inflammation regardless of the surface area of contact or the type of material used in making the pontic, the shift in emphasis has been towards accessibility and ease of cleansing rather than the actual design (Figures 5.58 and 5.59). It is possible that many patients prefer the saddle pontic because it feels and looks like a tooth (Figures 5.60 and 5.61).

Indications and contraindications

Of all the procedures in restorative dentistry, the acid-etch technique has been one of the most influential in giving credence to the term 'painless dentistry'. Due to the simplicity and effectiveness of the technique, it has applications in virtually every branch of dentistry and, most importantly, in the treatment of the young patient with traumatized, disfigured or missing front teeth. Broken teeth may be built up to their original form with tooth-coloured resins which adhere tenaciously to the clean, etched surface of enamel. Missing teeth could be replaced by directly bonding an artificial tooth (or even the patient's own) to the abutment teeth. The attractiveness of such simple techniques is undoubtedly the low cost and the great convenience in its execution. Very little or no tooth preparation, other than the cleaning and etching of the enamel surfaces, is required. All this enhances the patient's confidence in the dentist and acceptance of the dentistry being performed. Cultivation of such admirable attitudes is extremely important because, although the procedures are not as arduous as those for conventional bridgework, the patient's full cooperation must nevertheless be obtained if a satisfactory result is to be achieved.

Furthermore, unless the patient is willing to attend at regular intervals to have the bridge (and indeed the whole mouth) examined, it would be unwise to proceed with any form of fixed bridge-

[*contd on page 114*]

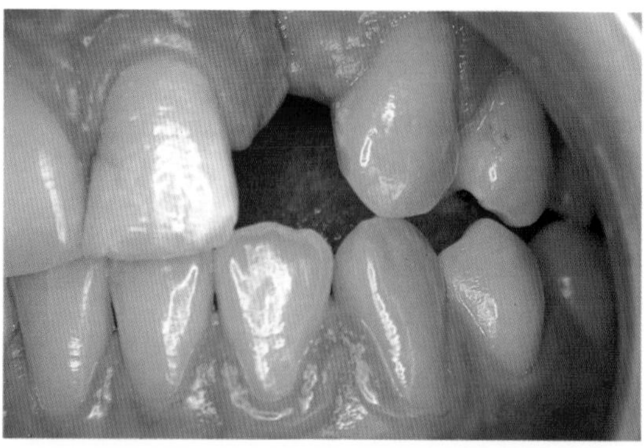
a

Figure 5.52

This patient with a cleft palate required a resin-bonded bridge to replace a missing upper left lateral incisor. (a) The preoperative state;

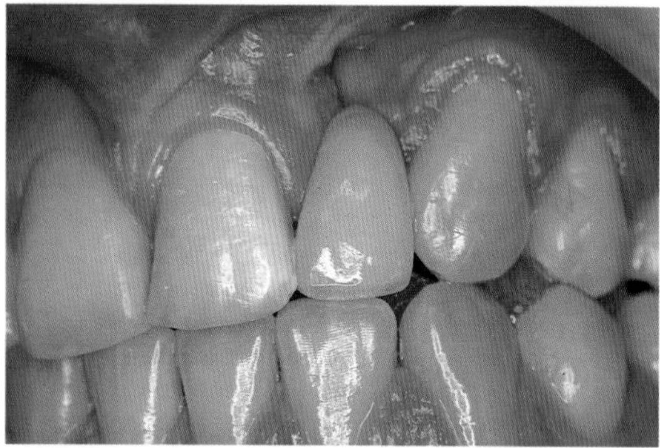
b

(b) the completed bridge in place;

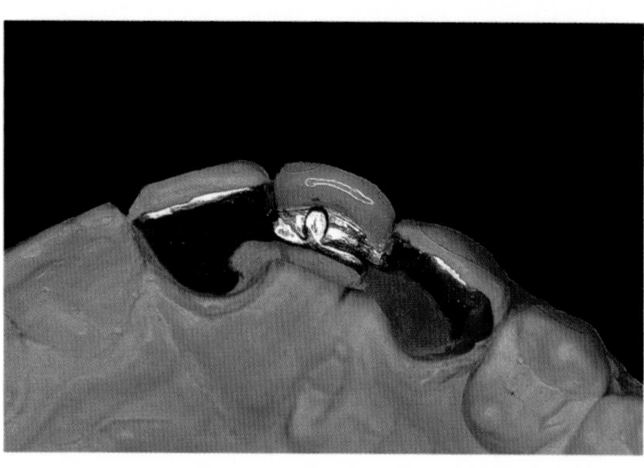
c

(c, d) the design incorporates a movable joint placed within the lateral incisor pontic. (Courtesy of Dr P.D. Cheshire.)

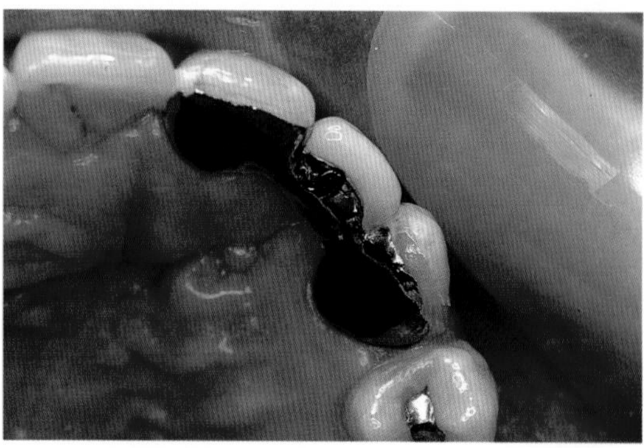
d

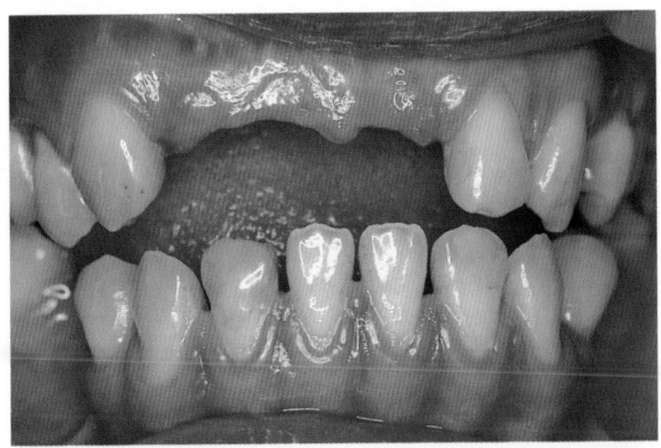

a

Figure 5.53

(a) Long-span bridges posed particular problems in alignment of the distant abutment teeth.

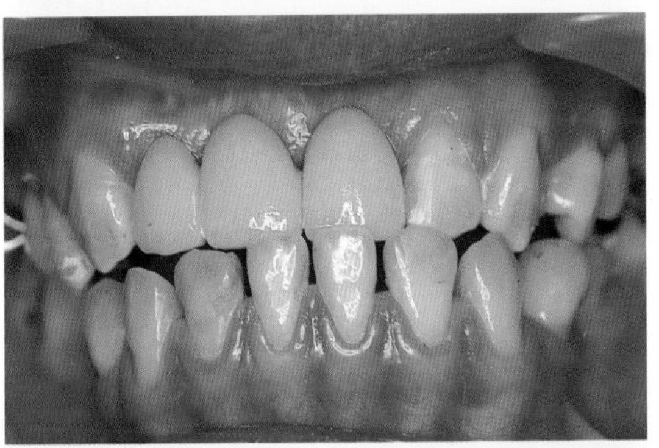

b

(b) This bridge spanning the upper left canine and right canine and first premolar has been split between the central incisor pontics with a movable joint attached to the lingual aspect of the mesial marginal ridges (c).

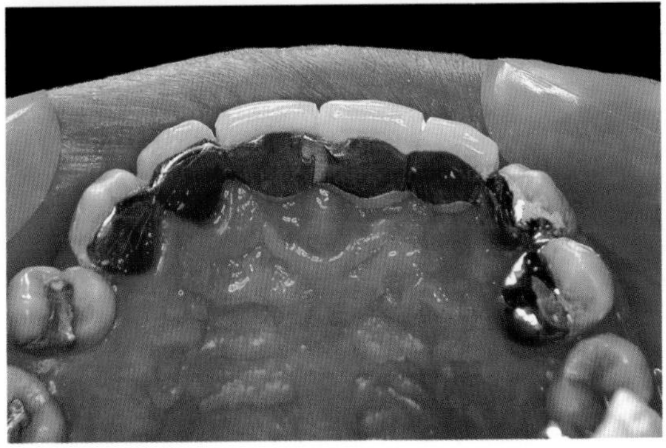

c

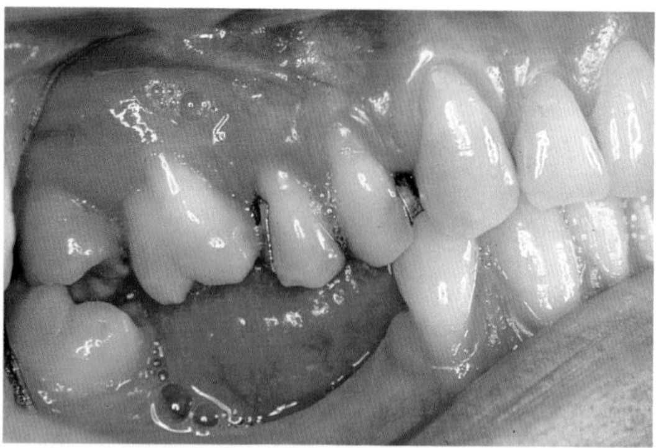

Figure 5.54

(a) Another case showing the length of span required between the lower right first premolar and second molar.

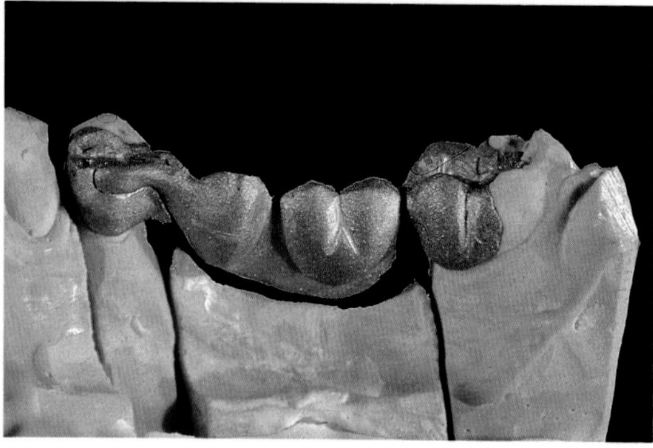

(b) Laboratory casting to show the movable joint situated on the distolingual aspect of the lower right first premolar.

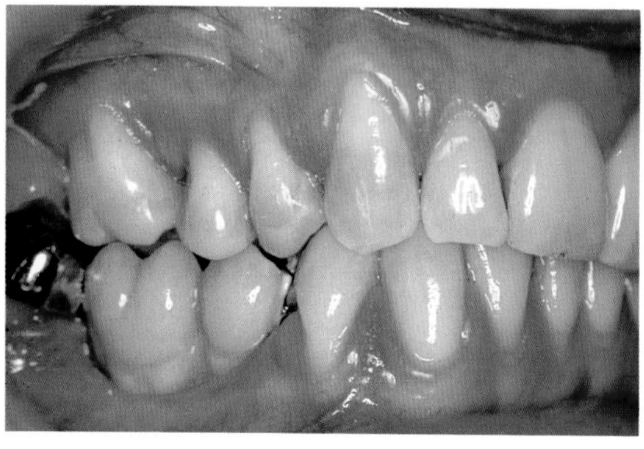

(c) The completed bridge in place. (Courtesy of Dr A.C. Shortall, with the kind permission of A.E. Morgan Publications Ltd.)

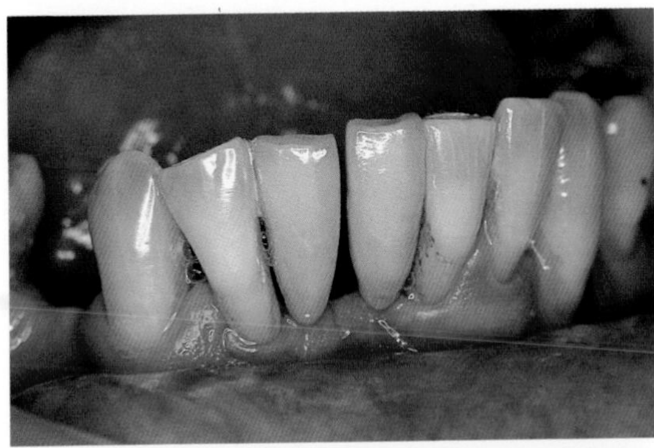

Figure 5.55

Two cantilever bridges replacing the lower central incisors with dome-shaped pontics with minimal tissue contact. (a) Labial view;

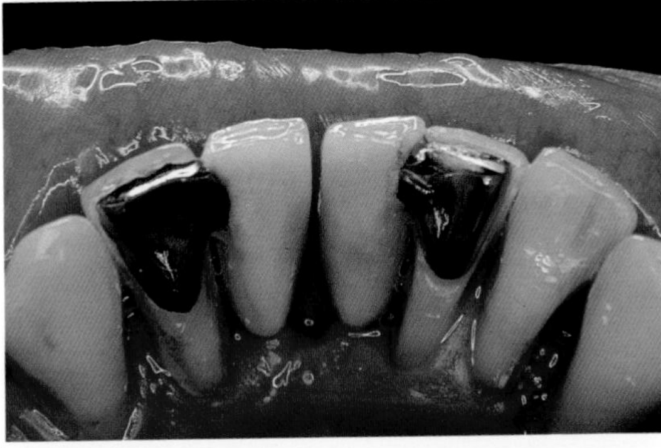

(b) lingual view.

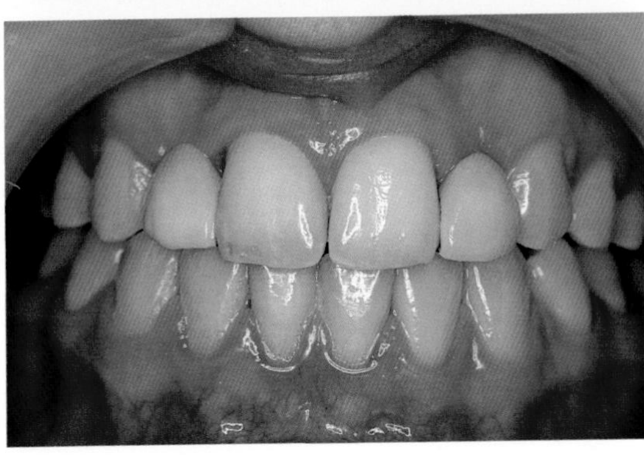

Figure 5.56

Cantilever bridges replacing the upper right and left lateral incisors with modified ridge lap pontics. (a) Labial view;

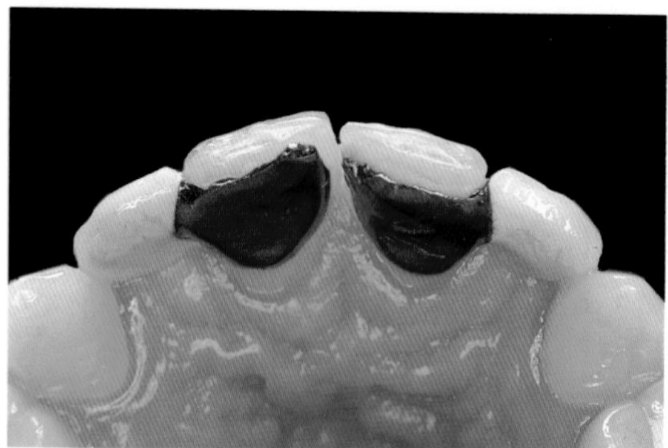

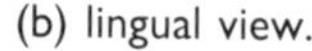

(b) lingual view.

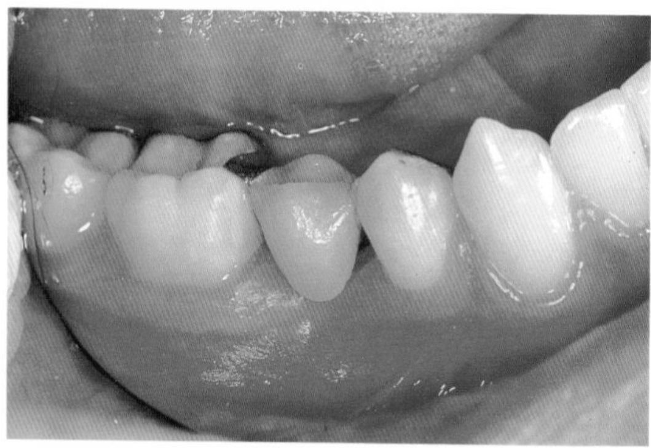

Figure 5.57

Fixed–fixed bridge replacing lower right premolar with modified ridge lap pontic. (a) Buccal view;

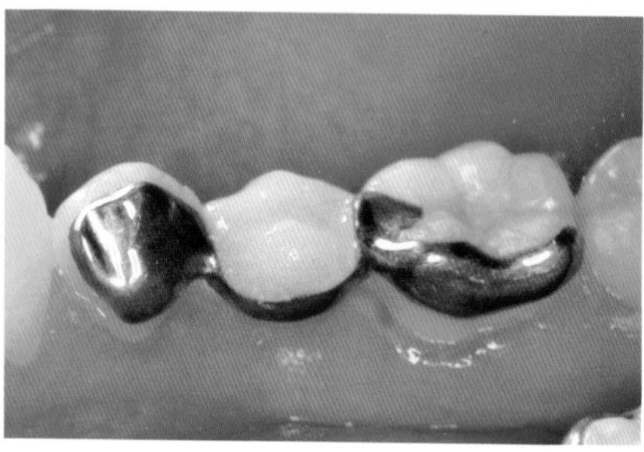

(b) lingual view.

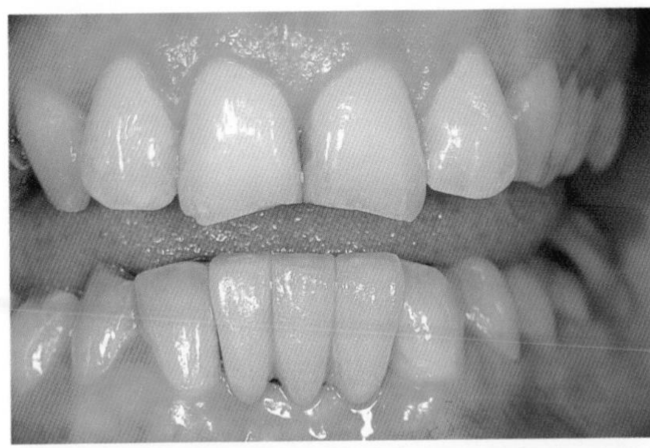

Figure 5.58

Poorly conceived, saddle-type pontic which would make cleaning difficult. (a) Labial view of pontic comprising three lower incisor teeth.

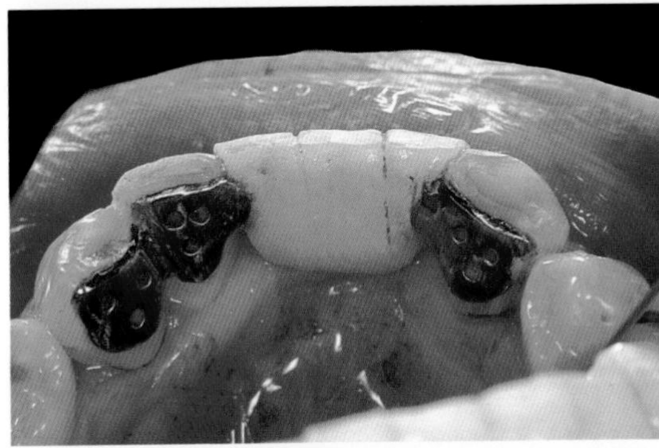

(b) Lingual view showing gross mucosal contact area.

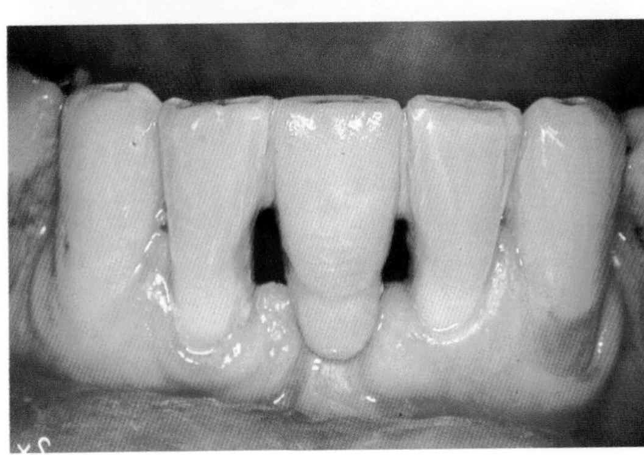

Figure 5.59

Well-designed, saddle-type pontic with wide embrasure spaces to facilitate cleaning. (Courtesy of Dr B.G. Tidmarsh.) (a) Labial view;

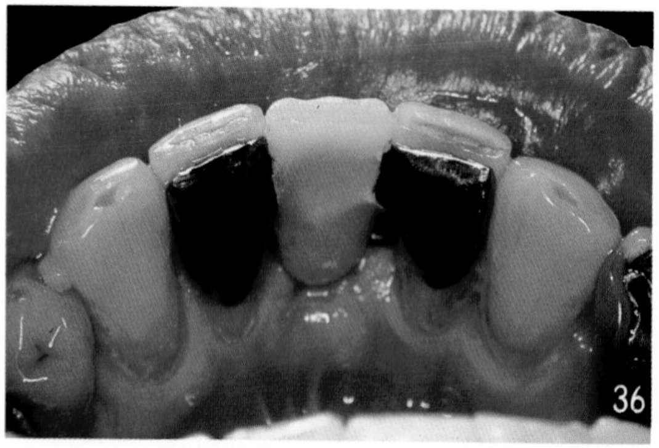

(b) lingual view.

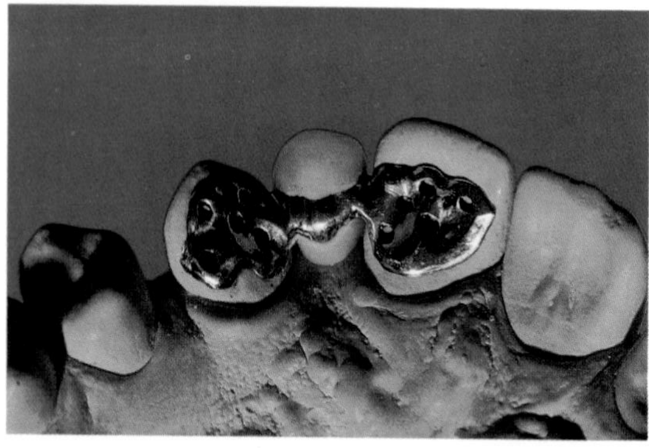

Figure 5.60

An example of a well-made, saddle-type pontic. (a) Lingual view showing bridge located on plaster cast.

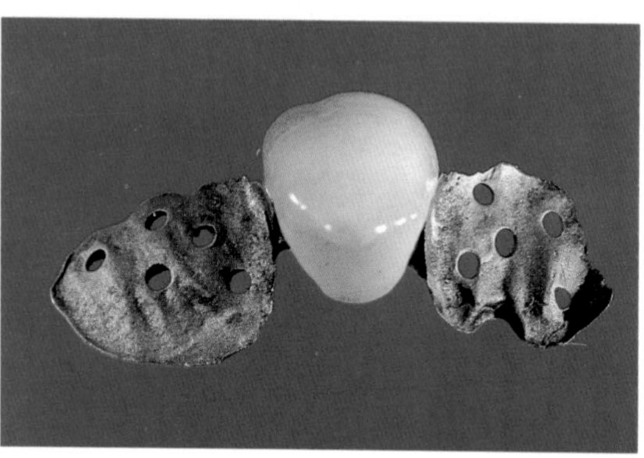

(b) Undersurface of porcelain pontic showing the extent of tissue contact inherent in this design.

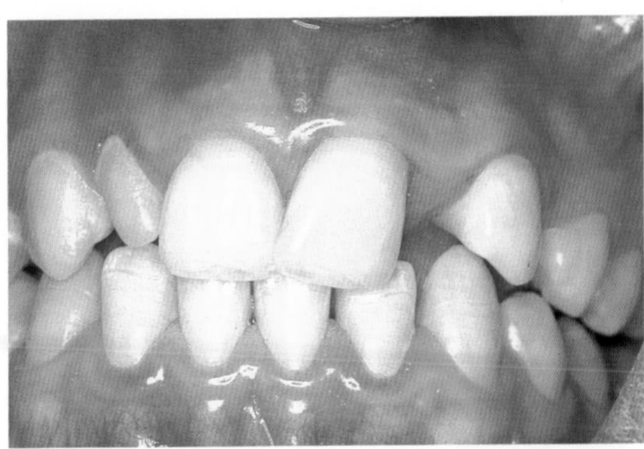

Figure 5.61

A saddle-type pontic comes closest to mimicking a natural tooth crown, and this example of a fixed–fixed bridge shows a well-made porcelain pontic replacing a missing upper left lateral incisor. (a) Preoperative appearance;

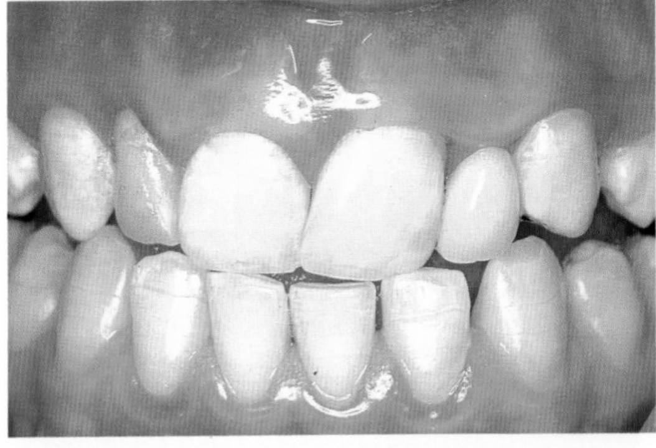

(b) bridge in place;

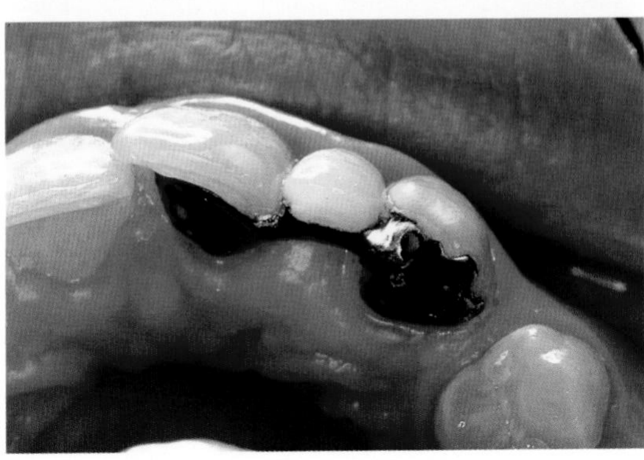

(c) incisal aspect.

work. With resin-bonded bridges, the first year is critical because most clinical studies have shown that the incidence of failure is greatest at this time.

During the recall appointments, the patient's oral hygiene can be monitored, the occlusion checked and the margins of the retainers examined for signs of resin breakdown and leakage which could lead to the development of caries and loss of attachment (debonding) of the retainer. The experience and information gained from these recall appointments can only contribute to a greater understanding of the performance of resin-bonded bridges—after all, these bridges are still undergoing development and evolution.

The danger with any seemingly simple technique is, however, the overconfidence that often arises. The practitioner may feel tempted to extend its application into difficult situations without giving due thought to possible complications. At present, resin-bonded bridges should not be looked at as a complete substitute for traditional bridgework (fixed prosthodontics). Rather, in selected cases these bridges may well provide a viable and acceptable alternative to 'conventional' methods.

Reasons for replacing missing teeth

There are three main reasons for such replacement: (1) aesthetics; (2) function; and (3) prevention.

Aesthetics

Aesthetics ('esthetics' in the USA) is a grandiloquent term to describe, in a vague sort of way, the pleasing appearance of a person's dentition. It provides the impetus which brings a patient to see a dentist in the first instance. To some patients this may be the supreme concern; therefore, disappointment is great when expectations are not fulfilled. The problem is usually confined to anterior teeth or the upper premolars. With the rapid reduction in the incidence of dental caries in many countries, 'aesthetic' or 'cosmetic dentistry' has become the prime 'practice builder'.

Function

The term 'function' generally refers to the 'ability to eat', and is often manifest in cases where two or more juxtaposed teeth are missing in one of the posterior quadrants of the dental arch, rendering that side of the mouth virtually non-functional. Yet, it is surprising how efficiently some patients can eat even with several teeth missing and, in this respect, Kayser (1981) has developed the concept of the 'shortened dental arch' where sufficient mandibular stability and occlusal function can exist with at least four 'occlusal units', especially if these are in a symmetrical position. However, others consider the deprivation of even a single molar tooth to be a physical handicap.

The loss of one tooth, especially an incisor, can affect speech quite markedly. The degree of impediment varies greatly from person to person and also depends largely on the type of occlusion present and on other anatomical and physiological factors that influence speech. Actors, teachers and politicians lose their stature if deprived of both speech and a pleasant mien, and so, obviously, in these and similar professions the replacement of any missing teeth is of paramount importance. Allied to the problem of speech when teeth are missing is a problem that is peculiar to wind instrument players. The term 'embouchure' refers to the manner in which the lips are applied to the mouthpiece of a wind instrument in order to produce tone. The circumoral muscles and the tongue play an important role in forming the 'embouchure', but they must function against the anterior teeth if the appropriate stream of air for a mellifluous sound is to be produced. Nixon (1963) has observed that 'professional musicians are usually sensitive individuals, almost always tending to be perfectionists and any circumstance which upsets their usual standard of play can produce a great deal of mental upset and lack of self-confidence which is reflected in their playing'. The great difficulty here will be the replacement of missing teeth with a bridge that is accurately contoured to allow the patient to adopt the accustomed 'embouchure' for his or her instrument.

Prevention

The loss of a tooth or teeth may result in the deterioration of the other teeth by virtue of the following:

1 The overeruption of an opposing tooth which may cause undesirable occlusal interferences, poor approximal contacts, periodontal breakdown and loss of bony support.
2 Drifting and tilting of the teeth mesial and distal to the space which may give rise to loss of approximal contacts, food stagnation and caries. Periodontal pocketing may be the direct consequence of food packing or the indirect result of occlusal derangement and un-favourable masticatory forces being applied to the teeth.

The placement of a bridge may prevent the unacceptable breakdown of the remaining dental structures.

Advantages of resin-bonded bridges

Minimal tooth preparation

With the falling caries rate in most societies and with the increasing incidence of children and young adults possessing a full set of decay-free teeth, it would seem reckless and irresponsible to grind away sound tooth tissue. At least 1.5–2.0 mm of tooth tissue needs to be removed in a standard aesthetic full crown preparation. In young teeth with large pulp chambers, this may be a hazardous procedure with the ever-present danger of pulpal irritation or, worse, a frank pulp exposure. Some teeth, especially the lower incisors, are unsuitable for conventional crown preparations because of their slenderness. Understandably, most dentists are reluctant to cut such teeth.

Expediency

With resin-bonded bridges, due to the minimal tooth preparation, there is little need to provide temporary (provisional) crowns other than for aesthetic reasons; there is also no necessity to perform any gingival retraction before taking an impression for working casts. With reduced chairside time and number of visits necessary for completion, the overall cost of the treatment is much less (although there may be great variation in dental laboratory charges). It has been estimated that the 'cost ratio' between resin-bonded and conventional bridges is in the region of 1:2–1:4 in favour of the resin-bonded bridge, given a bonding expectancy of 5 years.

The length of any treatment session is, of course, influenced by the amount of tooth preparation carried out and by the experience of the operator. On average, a dentist may be expected to spend 40–60 minutes on each session to a maximum of three sessions. Setting times of the various impression and luting materials used might be considered influential in prolonging treatment times, but in fact have been found to have only a negligible effect (Creugers and van't Hof, 1987).

No specialized training required

Provided the practitioner is versed with the general principles of crown and bridgework, and occlusal relationships, no special skills are required for this technique. Therefore, the scope of treatment options offered in a non-specialist general practice can be expanded, with increased benefit to the patients.

Convertibility

By virtue of their design, minimal preparation on the teeth and finite bond strengths of current resins, resin-bonded bridges are self-limiting in their potential destructiveness compared with full-coverage crown retainers in conventional bridgework. Therefore, should a resin-bonded bridge fail, for whatever reason, it would be possible to 'upgrade' to a conventional bridge without detriment to the health of the abutment teeth (which would be left relatively intact) or the periodontium. The converse, of course, is not feasible.

Acceptance by the patient

Any technique which involves the minimum of 'injections and drilling' is bound to find favour with patients. Even with the hesitant and suspicious patient, confidence can be cultivated and enhanced more easily than with conventional bridgework, because the technique is so much less arduous and expensive. However, it is important that the patient is made fully aware of the limitations of resin-bonded bridges.

Disadvantages of resin-bonded bridges

High failure rate

The high failure rate of resin-bonded bridges, when compared with that of conventional bridges, is arguably the main reason for deterring many dentists from offering this service to their patients.

Aesthetics

Discrepancies in pontic widths, soft tissue loss (Figures 5.62 and 5.63) and malpositioned abutments (Figure 5.64) are much more difficult to correct. In conventional bridgework, allowances can be made and the discrepancies compensated for by a combination of tooth preparation and astute laboratory craftsmanship.

Occlusal interferences

Consequent on these bridges being mostly retained by lingually (palatally) placed metal flanges and being bonded on to etched enamel, it is often not possible to reduce the abutment teeth sufficient to allow for the thickness of the metal while preserving the required surface of enamel. As a result, occlusal interferences may be created where none existed previously. This is a frequent problem when the upper anterior arch is involved. Also, with overcontouring caused by the presence of flanges on the abutment teeth, there may be a tendency towards increased plaque retention.

No trial period possible

Occasionally, for aesthetic, functional or periodontal reasons, it may be desirable to fit bridges temporarily with a form of 'non-setting' cement. Then, after a period of probation, and if all is well and the patient satisfied, the bridge can be removed easily and recemented with a 'permanent' cement. Such a procedure, although not impossible with resin-bonded bridges, is certainly not practical.

Indications for resin-bonded bridges

The most appropriate occasions for prescribing a resin-bonded bridge are the following:

1. In young patients with sound abutment teeth but with large pulp chambers.
2. In patients who may not wish to endure extensive crown and bridge procedures.
3. For patients who may otherwise be unable to afford conventional bridge treatment. The saving is in the reduced chairside time.
4. Where there is a reluctance, on the part of both dentist and patient, to cut sound teeth, or where teeth are unsuitable for preparations, eg the lower incisors or root-filled teeth.
5. In medically 'at-risk patients' where prolonged dental procedures may be undesirable, or where antibiotic cover is required every time any form of 'traumatic' dentistry is carried out.
6. As an interim bridge, eg following periodontal surgery. The mucosa is allowed to recover full health before commencing conventional bridgework.
7. As a space maintainer, periodontal or orthodontic retention splint (Figures 5.65 and 5.66). The cast metal splints are the strongest in this respect.
8. In occlusal therapy where new guide planes may be created on the lingual surfaces of the flanges (Thayer and Doukoudakis, 1981). These may be individual units (Figure 5.67) or part of the bridge framework.
9. In partial dentures, where resin-bonded metal flanges can be used to create retentive or supportive surfaces for denture clasps or rests (Figure 5.68).

Contraindications for resin-bonded bridges

There are situations where resin-bonded bridges are not recommended. Some of these are discussed

[*contd on page 123*]

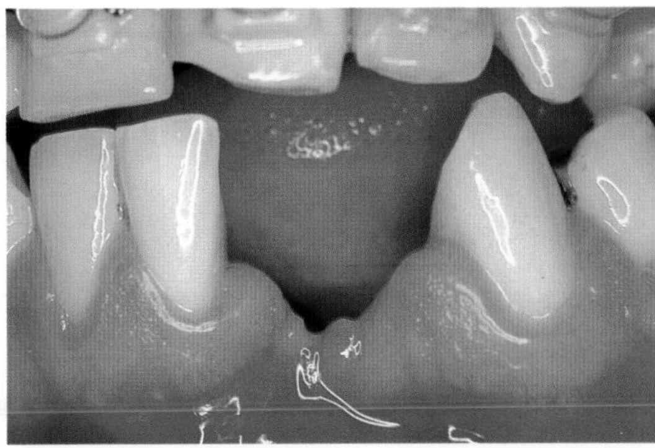

Figure 5.62

(a) Excessive soft tissue and bone loss has resulted in a collapsed ridge.

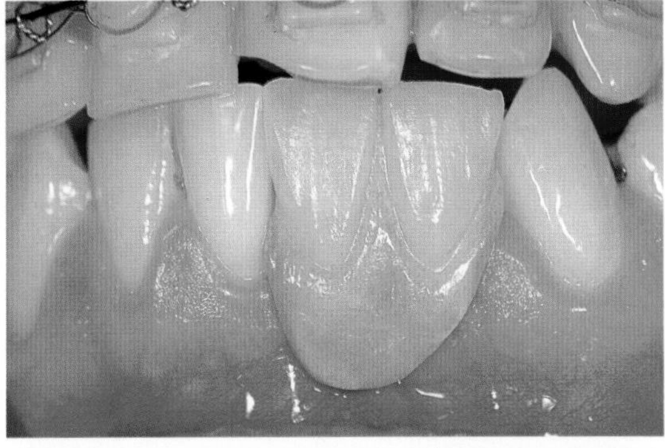

(b) Filling in the defect with pink porcelain on the pontic in this instance was aesthetically acceptable to the patient, but may pose problems with bridge hygiene.

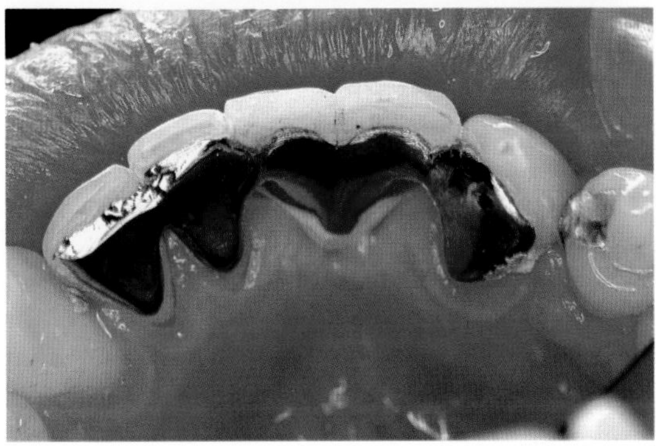

(c) Lingual aspect of the fixed–fixed bridge.

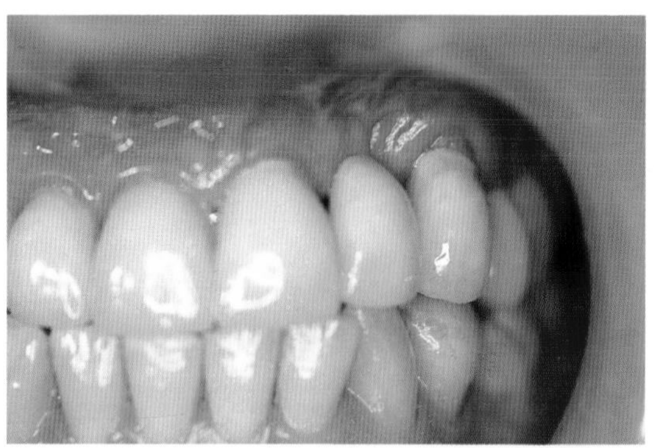
a

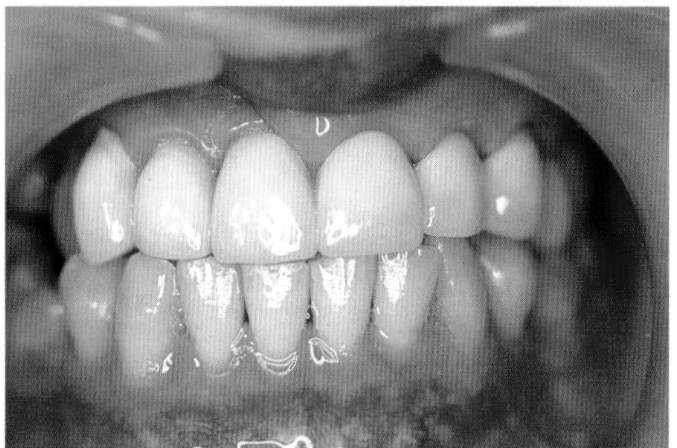
b

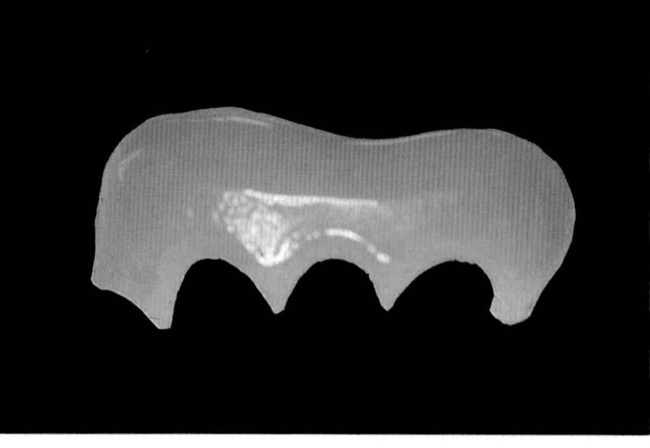
c

Figure 5.63 (a–c)

(a) Small discrepancies in the gingivae and mucosa of the ridge may be masked with a pink acrylic slip (b,c) which can be removed by the patient for cleaning.

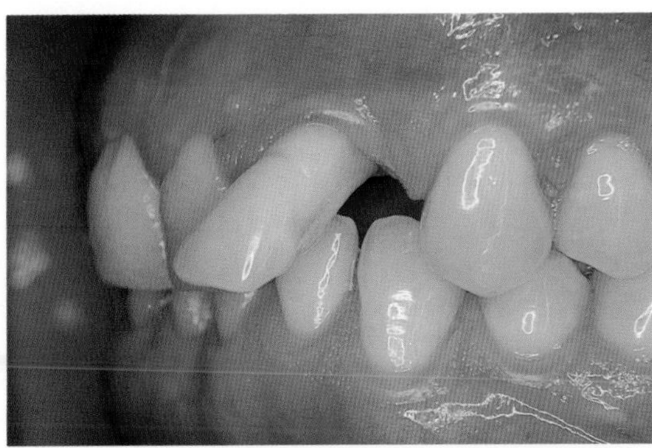

Figure 5.64

A malpositioned tooth is unlikely to be suitable as a bridge abutment.

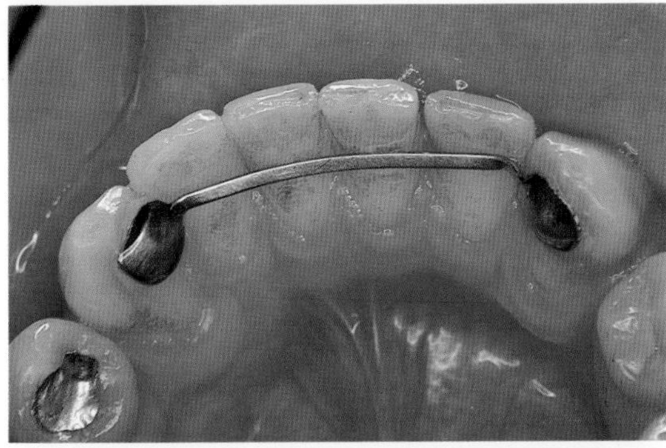

Figure 5.65

A resin-bonded, orthodontic arch retainer using etched metal pads on the lower canines supporting a lingual bar. (Courtesy of Mr J. Page.)

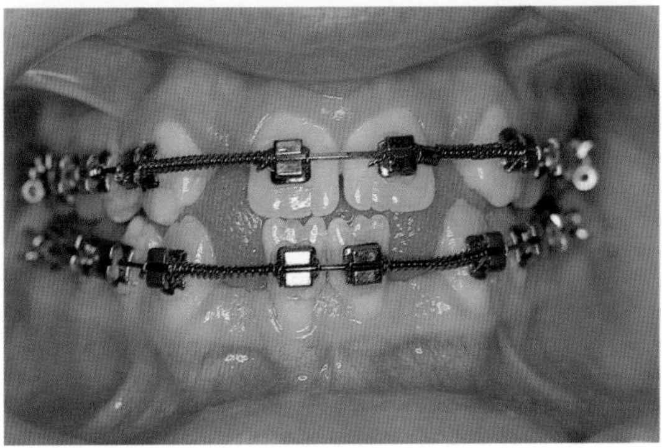

Figure 5.66

Resin-bonded bridges may be used in conjunction with orthodontic treatment to improve aesthetics and maintain the stability of the dental arches. (a) This patient is a young female with congenitally missing upper and lower lateral incisors. The upper and lower arches have fixed appliances to correct overcrowding.

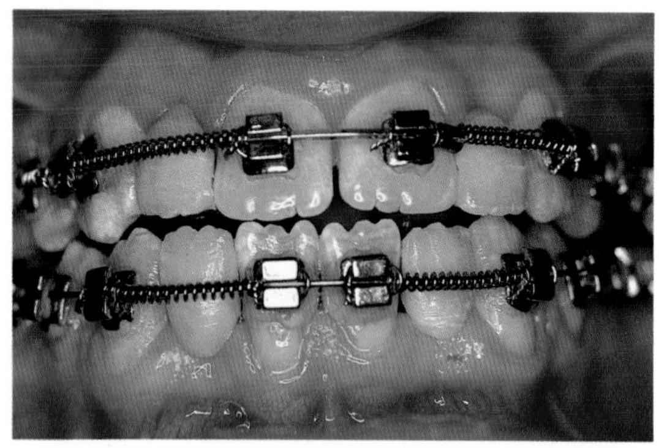

(b) The orthodontic treatment has been successful and now fixed–fixed, resin-bonded bridges have been placed in the position of the missing lateral incisors.

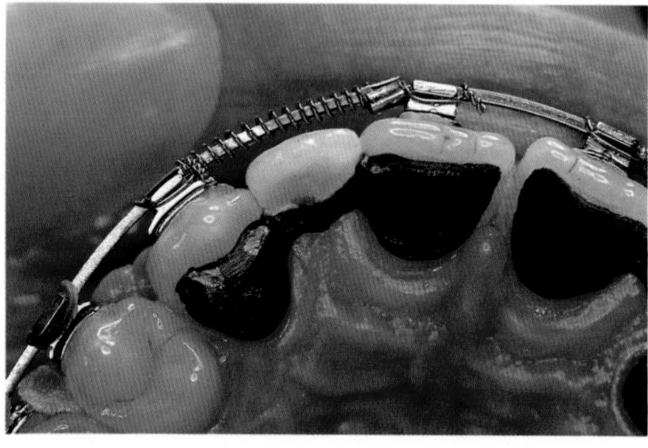

(c) Palatal view of upper right bridge.

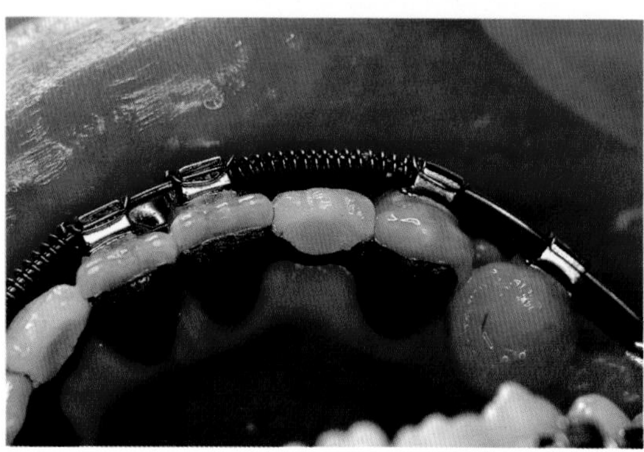

(d) Lingual view of the lower right bridge. The orthodontic appliances were subsequently removed.

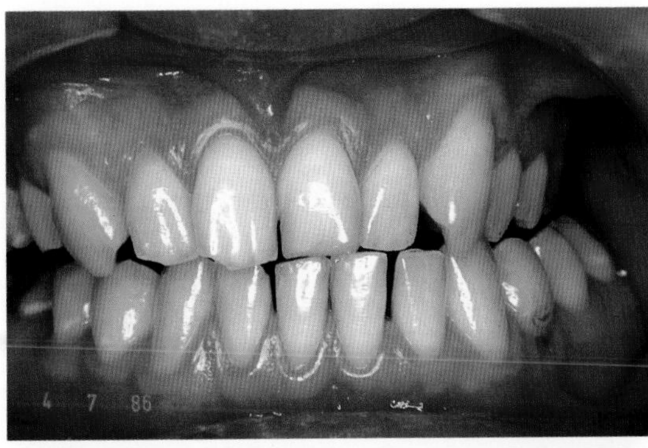

Figure 5.67

Resin-bonded metal pads may be used to create occlusal guidance planes. (a) Preoperative view shows lack of guidance contact between upper canines (cuspids) and opposing lower teeth.

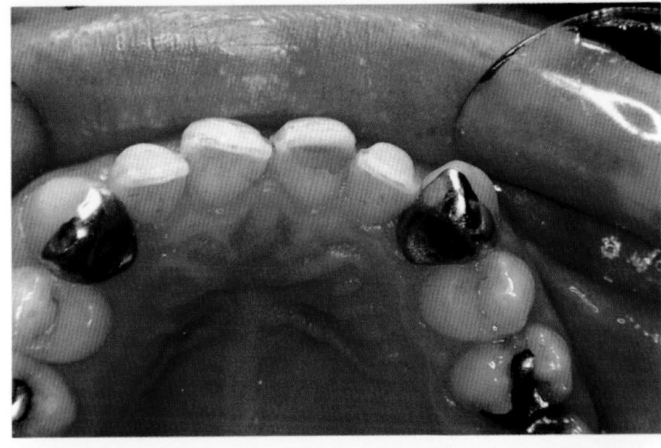

(b) Resin-bonded pads were placed on the upper canines.

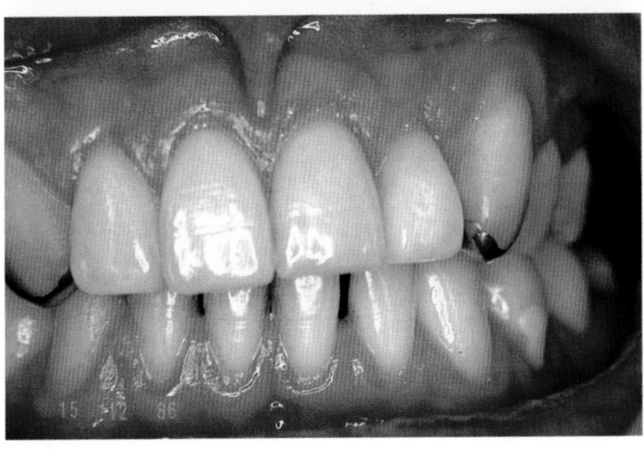

(c) Good contact has been achieved. (Courtesy of Mr P.D. Cheshire.)

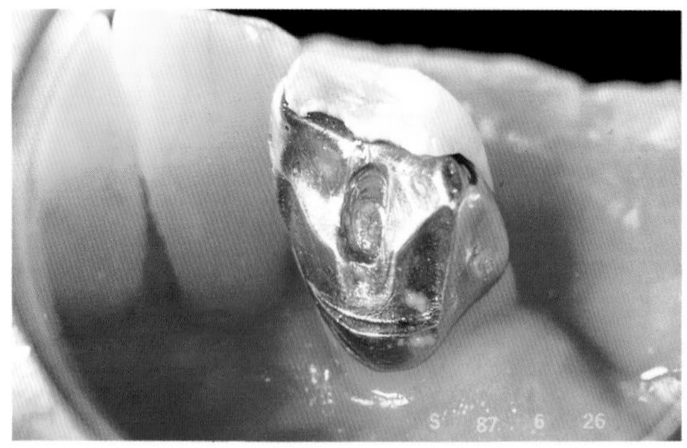

Figure 5.68

Resin-bonded metal flanges or pads may be used to support and retain removable prostheses (partial dentures). (a) Lingual view of flange showing milled surfaces and rest seats.

(b) Denture clasp in position. (Courtesy of Dr S.E. Northeast.)

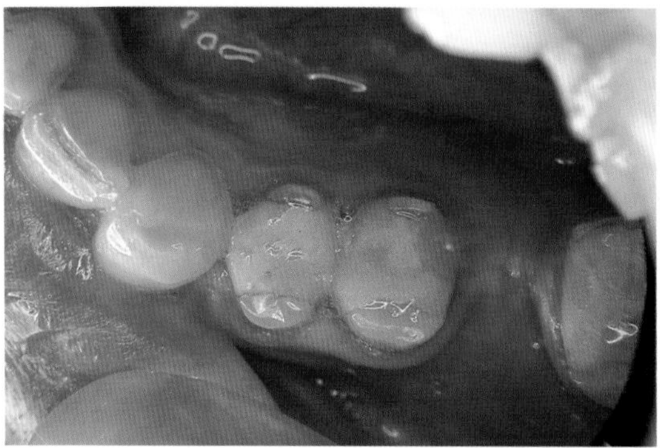

Figure 5.69

The small gap could have been successfully bridged with a resin-bonded appliance but for the poor quality of the abutment teeth, which have large and unsatisfactory composite resin restorations.

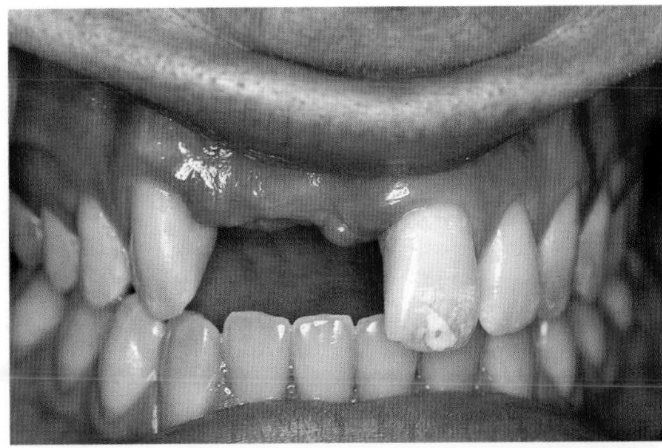

Figure 5.70

A discrepancy between the length of the saddle and the number of pontic units which can be fitted within it may pose aesthetic problems. (a) Preoperative state showing a fairly long saddle.

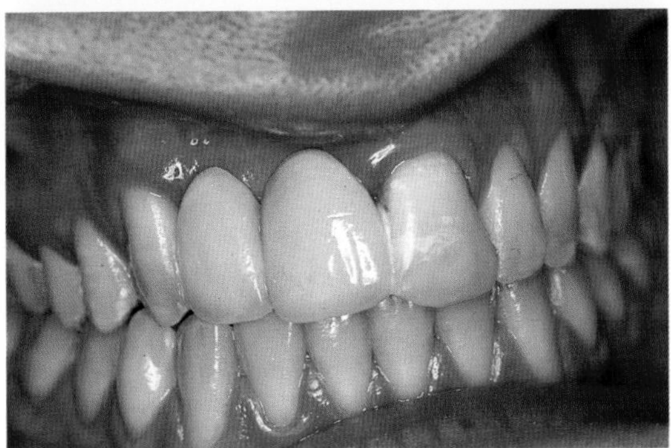

(b) The central and lateral incisor pontic units have been overcompensated, leading to a less than satisfactory result.

elsewhere, but it would be valuable to reiterate them if only to emphasize their importance:

1 Where there is insufficient or poor quality enamel for etching and bonding, eg very short clinical crowns, partially erupted teeth and extensively destroyed teeth caused by caries or previous restorations (Figure 5.69). Unfortunately, a high caries rate may often be at its peak in the under-21 age group for whom resin-bonded bridges may be the treatment of choice. Uncontrolled caries leads to the destruction of sound enamel which is essential to the success of these bridges.
2 Long-span bridges, ie those with more than two pontic units, may be unsuitable (see Figure 5.15). Generally, the longer the span of the pontic saddle, the greater will be the leverage and stress imposed on the tooth–resin–metal bonds.
3 Where there is a large discrepancy between the width of the saddle and the actual number of pontic units that can be fitted in to give a pleasant and balanced aesthetic result (Figure 5.70). This applies mainly to the anterior quadrant where this would be difficult to achieve because no gross tooth reduction is performed. In a conventional bridge, full crown preparations on the abutment teeth provide a greater leeway for the technician to create the desired effect. Similarly, where there is excessive soft tissue loss, even the artful deception of shaping the pontic or using tissue-coloured ('pink') porcelain which a skilled technician can produce may not realize the desired effect (see Figure 5.62). Smaller disparities affecting gingival tissues may be masked with a pink acrylic veneer or 'gum slip' which can be removed by the patient for cleaning (see Figure 5.63).

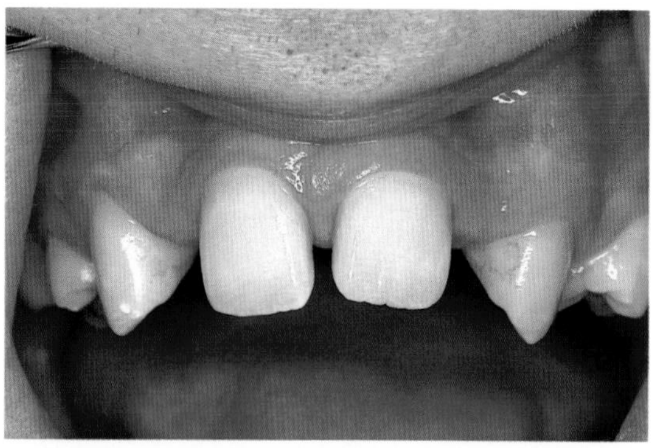

Figure 5.71

Simple orthodontic treatment may be carried out to achieve more space for the pontic. (a) Preoperative view: the upper lateral incisor saddles are too narrow for a good aesthetic result.

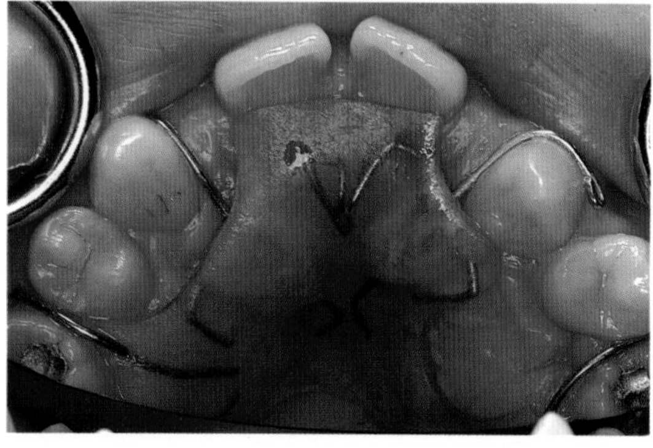

(b) A simple but effective orthodontic appliance was used to move back the canines.

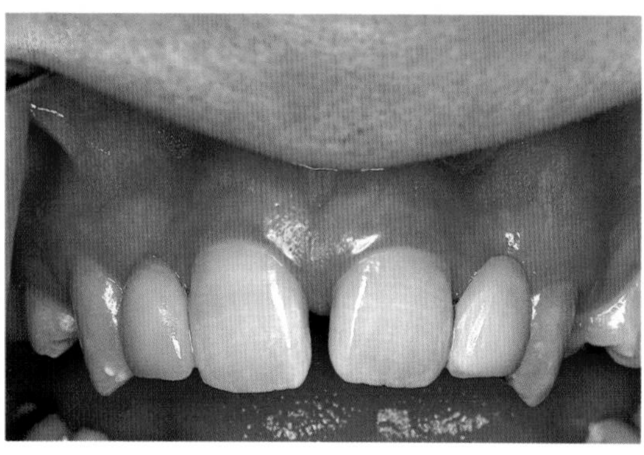

(c) Resin-bonded bridges in place. The small diastema between the upper central incisors has been preserved.

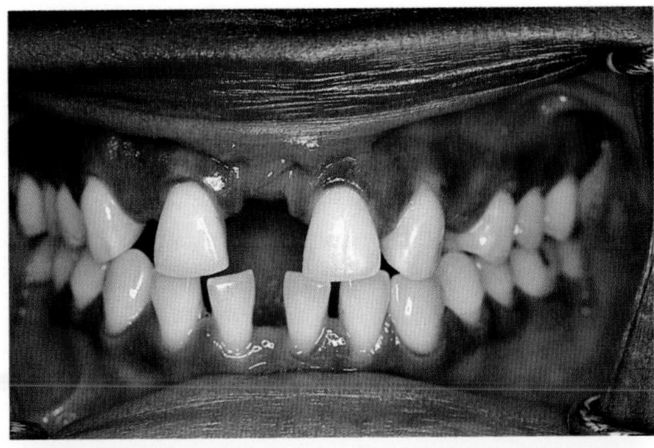

Figure 5.72

A wide median diastema may be effectively treated with cantilevered resin-bonded bridges. (a) Labial view: preoperative.

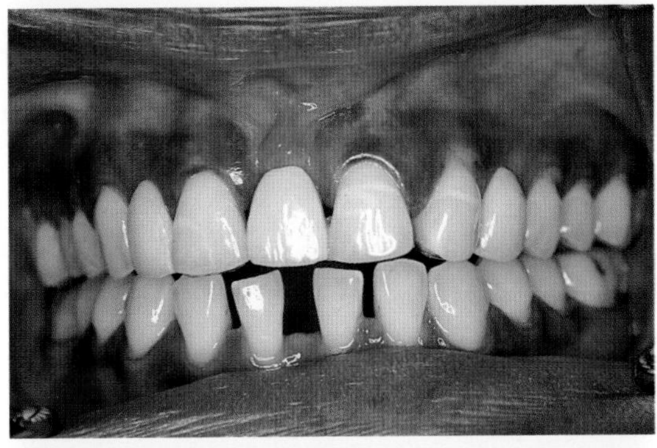

(b) Bridges in place: the effect of three 'central' incisors is not as distractive as might be feared. The lower diastema was left untreated.

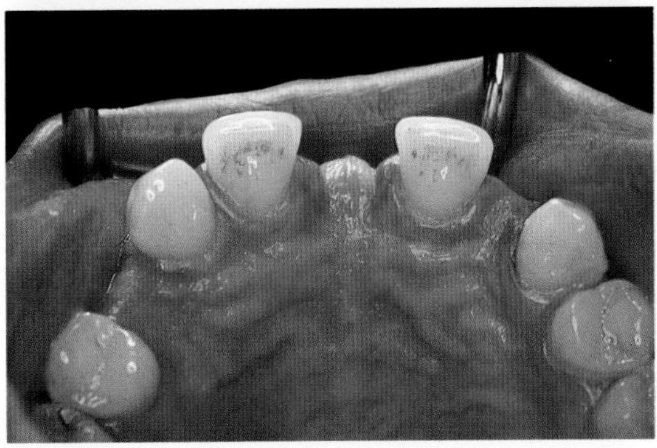

(c) Palatal view: preoperative.

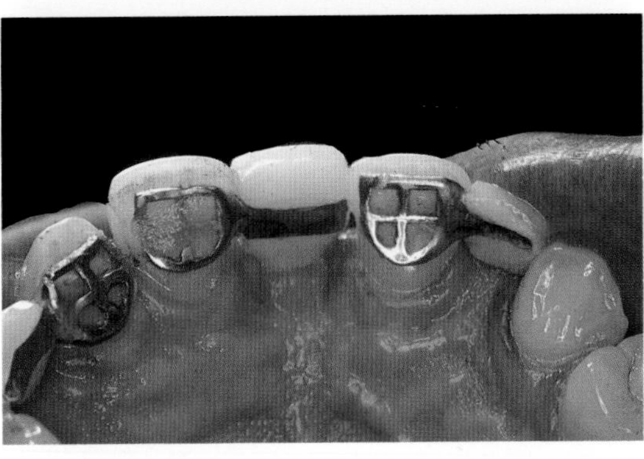

(d) Palatal view showing the three cantilever bridges of the 'Rochette' design.

4 Where there is insufficient occlusal clearance or heavy occlusal forces are present, eg in patients who suffer from bruxism. The patient with a deep overbite poses great difficulties, especially if an upper anterior bridge is contemplated.
5 Badly aligned, spaced teeth, or diastemas, may also present aesthetic problems. Ideally, as in conventional bridgework, some preliminary orthodontic intervention should be carried out (Figure 5.71). If this is not feasible, then, at least for badly tilted teeth, the problem is not as severe as for conventional bridgework where the integrity of the pulp may be in jeopardy due to the need for tooth preparations in 'parallel'. Provided a preliminary survey of the tilted abutment teeth is carried out, it may be possible to circumvent excessive undercuts without compromising retention. A cantilever bridge, with or without a palatal bar, may be the only solution to the problem of diastemas (Figure 5.72 and see Figure 5.5).
6 Patients indulging in violent sports are generally discouraged from having any form of bridgework, and a partial denture which can be removed during the sporting activity is usually prescribed. Bridgework is deferred until the patient finally retires from his or her sport. Presumably, the reason for this is to avoid financial embarrassment or irretrievable damage to the abutment teeth caused by injury. Constant visits to the surgery for reattachment of the dislodged bridge may prove exasperating for both dentist and patient. However, considering the 'self-limiting' characteristic of resin-bonded bridges, it may be argued that the convenience of having a secure resin-bonded bridge far outweighs the inconvenience of an occasional dislodgement, especially if a mouthguard could be worn during the physical activity. In this instance, the patient's wishes must be paramount but tempered by judicious advice.

Clearly, then, clinical success is greatly enhanced if there is a deliberate effort at selecting only those patients with features and characteristics conducive to bridgework in general and resin bonding in particular. Equally important is the collaboration with and empathy of a reliable and skilled dental technician or laboratory. The patient must be made aware of the limitations of such bridges which remain essentially in a state of development and evolution; likewise, the practitioner must be willing to offer some form of guarantee once the bridgework is undertaken should irrevocable failure occur.

6 Clinical procedures

Introduction

The special considerations of treatment planning for resin-bonded bridges must, of course, be part of the overall policy of meeting the demand of dental care—an objective defined as that care which is intended to establish the most effective dentition and level of oral health for the remainder of the patient's life through the minimum of treatment, while maintaining a proper balance between the dentist's responsibilities to individual patients and to the community as a whole.

At the preliminary visit, such general procedures as identifying the treatment required, stabilizing the dental condition, eg by removal of active caries, or constructing temporary appliances to provide acceptable appearance and function would be carried out. An assessment of the technical facilities available is also part of the initial procedure. Contemplation of the definitive treatment plan may then be made and discussed with the patient who, having been thus counselled and informed of the financial costs, would be much more appreciative of the efforts of the practitioner.

From discussions in the preceding chapters, it will be evident that all the important theoretical and clinical principles of conventional bridgework apply equally well to resin-bonded bridges. Due to the peculiar constraints of these bridges, case selection is stringent in terms of the patient's oral hygiene, occlusal relationships and suitability of abutment teeth. The patient should, at the outset, be told of the limitations of a resin-bonded bridge (in addition to its virtues); in particular, the patient's cosmetic expectations must be fully noted and the ability of the bridge to fulfil these requirements carefully assessed in case high hopes might be dashed. Previous photographs and records are most useful in this respect.

Occlusal examination, supplemented by occlusal records and study models, assists in the design of the most appropriate bridge. On the study models, a 'mock-up' of the proposed bridge can be made from stock denture teeth and pink wax, and can be given a trial in the mouth so that the patient has some idea of what the final result might be. Shade selection and prescription may also be carried out at this stage.

Tooth preparation

The various facets of tooth preparation for the stability and retention of the bridge have already been discussed in Chapter 5. Aesthetic and occlusal considerations feature prominently and may involve the partial removal of enamel, the creation of occlusal and cingulum rest seats, the provision of vertical parallel grooves or boxes on the approximal or lingual aspects of the tooth, the recognition of undercuts and paths of insertion, and the replacement of existing restorations which may be involved in the design. Although it might appear that the degree of precision required in tooth preparation for resin-bonded bridges is not the same as for conventional bridgework, a perfunctory approach is nevertheless likely to cause problems at the later stages.

A rubber dam may be applied for greater visibility and clarity of enamel modification. Friction-grip diamond burs are the main instruments used in tooth preparation. Their particular applications are listed here only as a general guide, and practitioners may have their individual preferences (Box F).

Impressions

The same degree of care should be used for impression-taking in resin-bonded bridges as is required in taking impressions for conventional fixed bridgework. The margins of the bridge tend to be supragingival in most cases, with the result that gingival retraction is not generally necessary and the technique is greatly simplified. The impression material should be syringed to reproduce all the features without being marred by air bubbles. Any accurate and stable impression material may be used according to the practitioner's preference, and may include the reversible hydrocolloids, polysulphides, polyethers or polyvinylsiloxanes (Figure 6.1).

Impressions for periodontal splints

For the construction of periodontal splints, the technique used in taking an impression of periodontally mobile teeth is slightly more tricky. The weight of the impression material, or even the momentum generated by injecting the viscous substance, can quite easily cause slight displacement of the mobile teeth, resulting in later problems in accuracy of fit and insertion of the finished splint. Here, the technique is first to immobilize the loose teeth by etching only the labial surfaces and bonding on a band of light-cure composite resin. Large interdental spaces should also be blocked out with wax. An impression of the lingual surfaces can then be taken safely and the temporary resin splint may be left in place until after the final metal splint has been bonded in place.

Occlusal records

If the technician receives sufficient information regarding the patient's jaw and tooth relationships, crowns and bridges can be made to such a high degree of precision that virtually no occlusal adjustments need be made on insertion in the mouth. This information is delivered by means of:

1 Accurate impressions and casts.
2 Proper articulator selection.
3 Detailed occlusal records.

The degree of care and effort in articulator selection and occlusal recording is generally related to the complexity of the case, and whether or not the patient's occlusion is to be reconstructed. By its very nature, a resin-bonded bridge is a simple appliance and not intended for complex occlusal

BOX F BURS FOR TOOTH PREPARATION

The following are suggested friction-grip diamond burs which may be used for tooth preparation in resin-bonded bridges:

Round	ISO No. 001/010, 001/018, 001/023; 1–2.3 mm diameter tip is for placing depth guide cuts before bulk enamel reduction; occlusal and cingulum rest seats
Flame	ISO No. 249/012, 249/016; 1.2–1.6 mm tip to reduce approximal enamel for maximum wrap-around of flange
Tapered	ISO No. 197/016; this round-ended tapered cylindrical diamond (1.6 mm tip) may be used to produce a small chamfer finishing line or create a curved guiding plane on the proximal surface next to the edentulous area
Tapered	ISO No. 170/018; this tapered cylinder with a 1.8 mm flat end is useful for producing cingulum rests, and also vertical groove or box preparations
Inverted cone	ISO No. 012/018; cingulum notches and rest seats may also be prepared with this short inverted cone diamond with a 1.8 mm tip

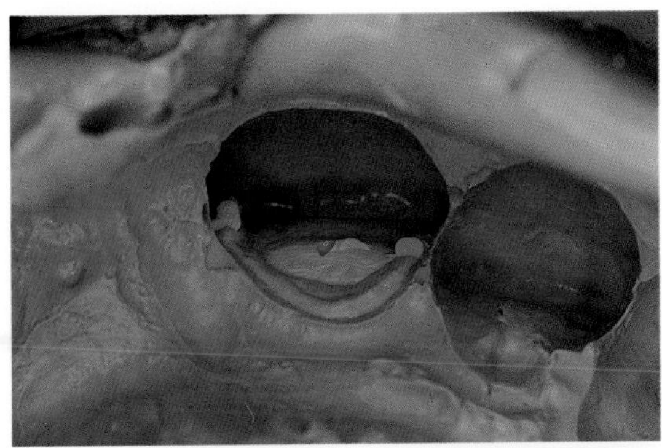

Figure 6.1

An impression made in a vinyl polysiloxane material.

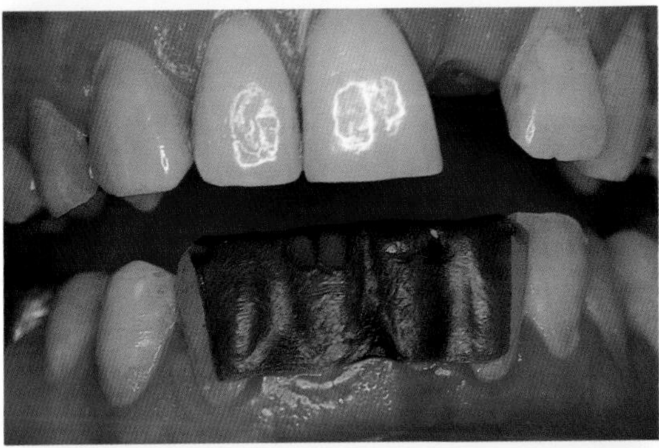

Figure 6.2

Occlusal adjustment of lower incisors before fabrication of bridge to replace upper left lateral incisor. (a) Occlusal indicator wax has been wrapped over lower incisor to define contacts with the upper right central incisor which is to carry the retainer flange.

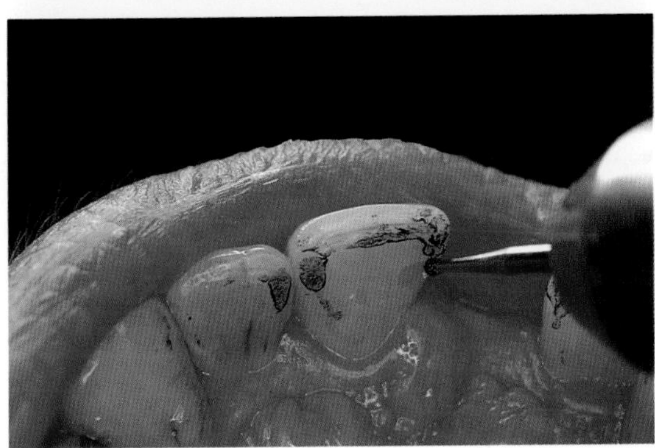

(b) Occlusal indicator tape has been applied to the upper right central incisor to mark the areas for occlusal reduction with a round diamond bur.

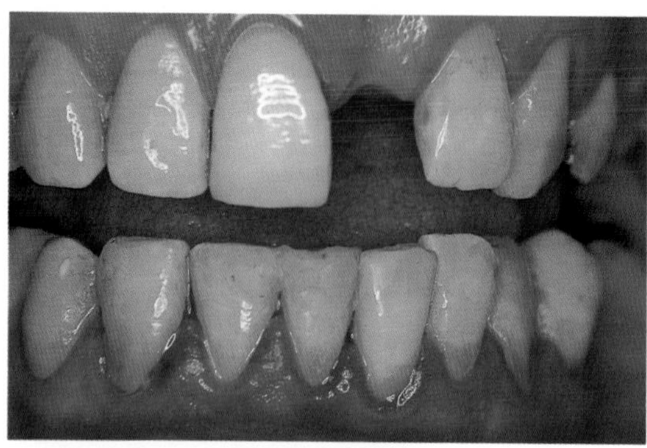

(c) The lower incisor edges have been built up with an etch-retained composite resin to re-establish occlusal contact.

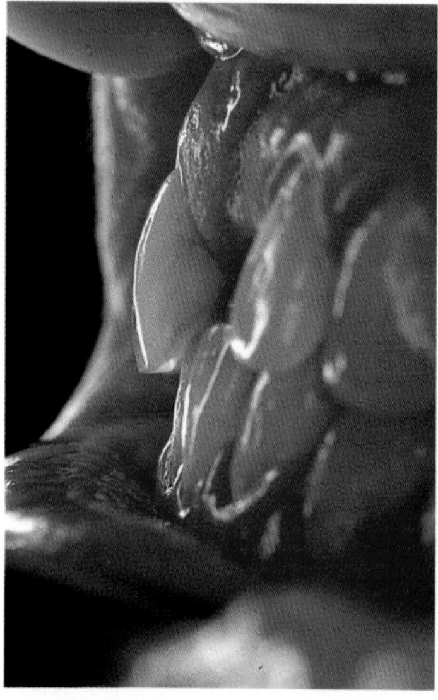

(d) Profile of the incisor relationship after occlusal reduction.

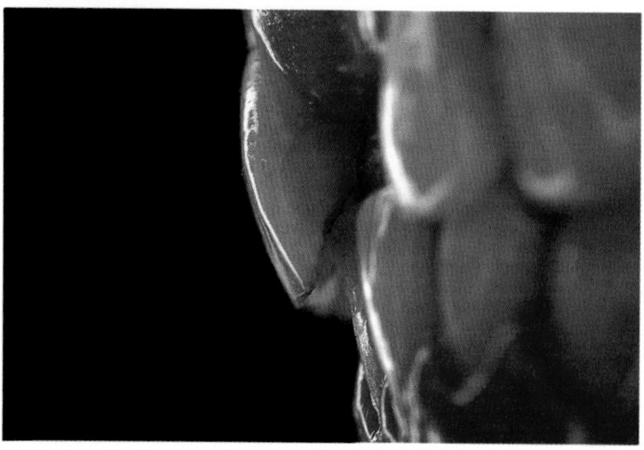

(e) The same view after re-establishing contact with an etch-retained composite resin. The composite resin is removed when the bridge is fitted.

rehabilitation. Therefore, most occlusal recording for resin-bonded bridges involves the registration of the *intercuspal position* (ICP).

With upper anterior bridges, the amount of occlusal adjustment (equilibration) may depend on the relationship of the mandibular to the maxillary anterior teeth, and whether or not the thickness of a lingual flange retainer may cause interference in ICP or disrupt anterior guidance.

No contact in ICP—open bite

If the ICP of the posterior teeth is stable and definite, then frequently the casts may be positioned manually or mounted on a plane line articulator, and occlusal registration is not essential.

Light contact in ICP—shallow anterior guidance

Where no extensive occlusal adjustment is envisaged then ICP registration, supplemented by lateral, protrusive and facebow transfer records, would be required. The casts may be mounted on a semi-adjustable articulator.

Moderate to steep anterior guidance

Where occlusal adjustment is contemplated for the restoration of the original anterior guidance pathways after fitting the bridge, the records obtained in the previous situation would be required. Occlusal adjustment may be approximate or relatively precise depending on the technique adopted:

1 The occlusion may be adjusted after cementation of the bridge by judicious 'grinding' with diamond burs and using articulating foil or tape, wax and shimstock to indicate uniform and balanced contacts.
2 Tooth reduction before bridge fabrication:
   (a) A small round diamond stone of diameter 1.0 mm (ISO No. 010) may be used initially to make depth cuts before bulk reduction with a small diamond wheel stone. If there is concern that, during the interim period when the bridge is being fabricated, the lower anterior teeth may overerupt into the space just created, they may be built up temporarily with an etch-retained, light-cured, composite resin (Figure 6.2); the resin is easily removed when the bridge is fitted.
   (b) In the simpler procedure of reducing the height of the opposing tooth, an accurate reduction can be performed on the working cast to suit the bridge under construction, so preserving the anterior guidance on each flange (Figure 6.3). A coping, which has a window framing the reduced area, can be made in a suitable acrylic or composite resin, or cast in scrap alloy. After the bridge has been bonded in place, the coping is positioned over the opposing tooth; the part protruding through the window can then be ground level with the coping to match the working cast. Anterior guidance can be recorded and set into an articulator by transferring the movements of the guide paths from the anterior teeth of the cast to the incisal guide block of a semi-adjustable articulator. The Whip-Mix, Denar Mark II, SAM and Hanau are examples of semi-adjustable articulators that provide a plastic incisal table suitable for moulding the incisal guidance in self-curing acrylic resin.

Intercuspal registration

Although wax 'bite' wafers are extensively used, the most assured record of the intercuspal position is one made with the teeth in contact with no intervening material to produce spurious contacts. However, lateral and protrusive records are almost invariably made in wax.

Temporary bridges (temporization)

Provided the preparations are only onto enamel, the patient should not experience any sensitivity. Sensitive exposed dentine may be covered with a thin film of a proprietary dentine-bonding agent or a light-cured, glass-ionomer cement.

If occlusal holding contacts have been removed on the opposing teeth, in order to make room for the thickness of the flange, then it may be necessary temporarily to re-establish the occlusal height of these teeth with an etch-retained, light-cured, composite resin while the bridge is being

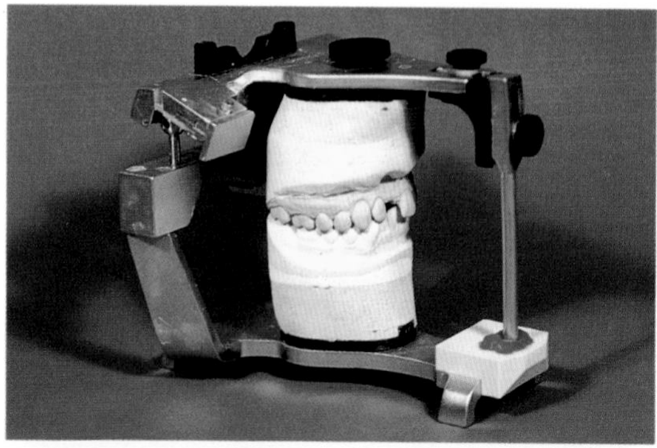

Figure 6.3

Laboratory-organized functional occlusion: (a) working models mounted on a semi-adjustable 'arcon' type articulator (Denar Mark II System, Denar Corporation).

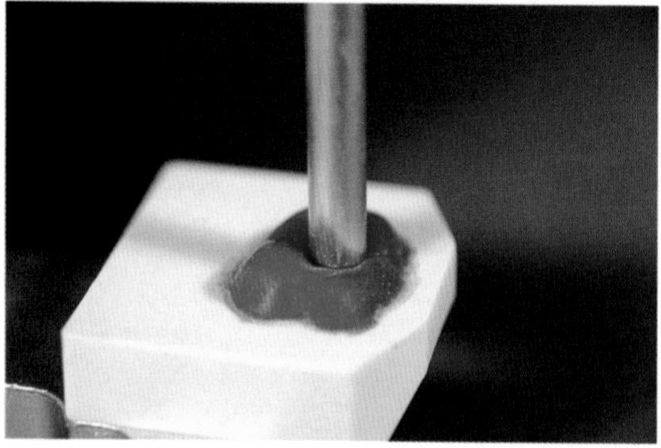

(b) Incisal guidance pathways moulded into an acrylic resin (Duralay Resin, Reliance Dental Manufacturing Co.) on the incisal guide block.

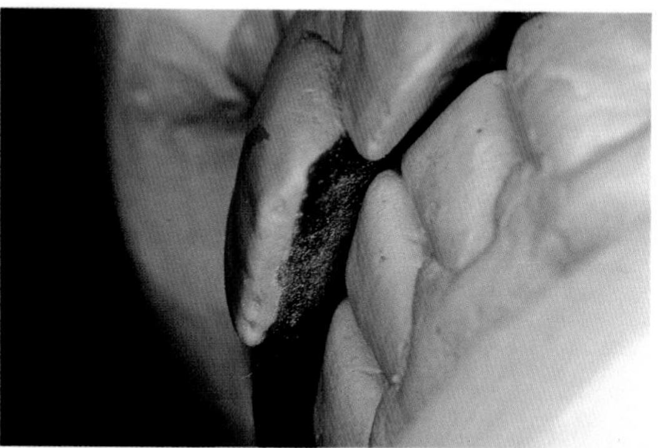

(c) The thickness of the flange as indicated by the wax-up interfering with the incisal guidance.

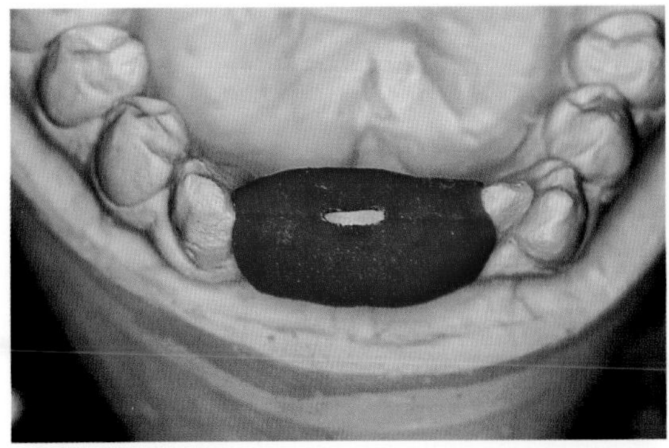

(d) Duralay coping with 'window' exposing the interference on the incisal edge.

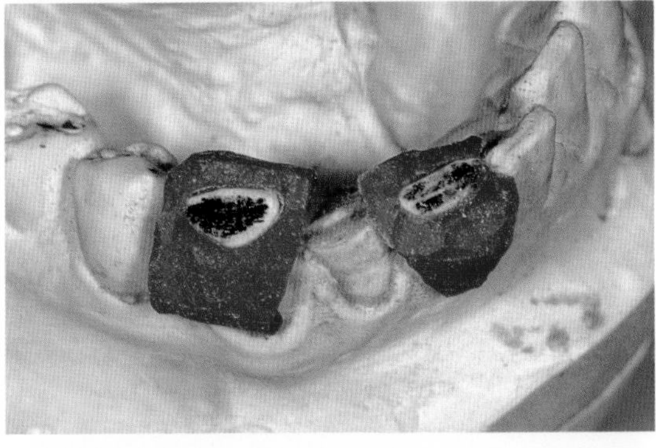

(e) A different case showing the coping window framing the interference area on the plaster cast which has been reduced by the laboratory technician.

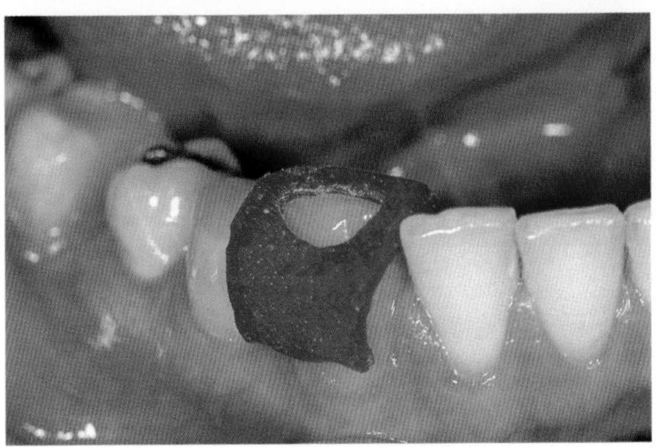

(f) Coping with window transferred to the mouth and placed over the tooth in question. Reduction of the incisal edge to the level of the window should thus correspond to the actual amount removed by the technician on the plaster cast.

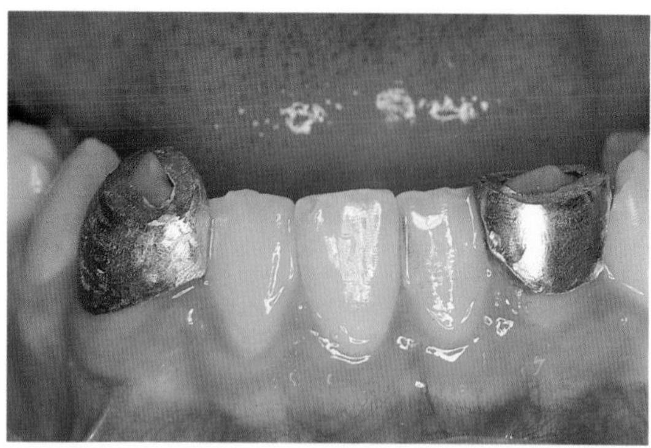

(g) Similar copings made with a silver alloy placed over the lower right canine and lower left lateral incisor.

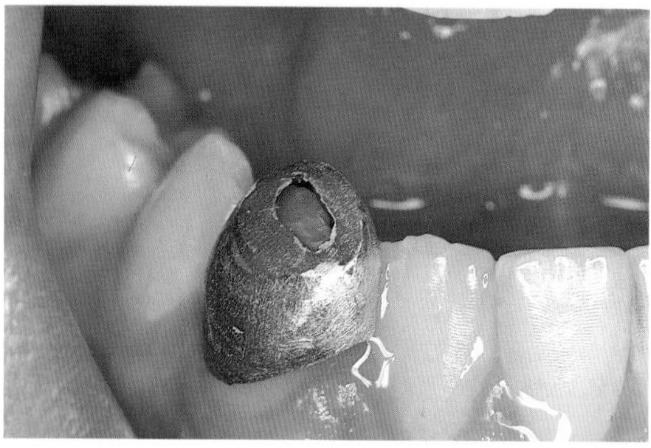

(h) Reduction of the lower right canine and

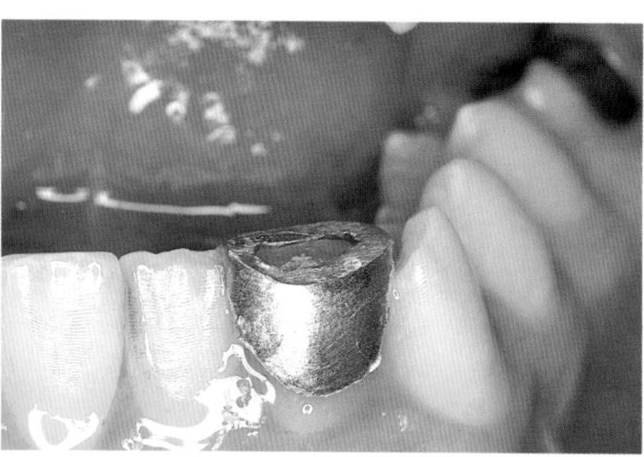

(i) lower left lateral incisor.

made; this is done to prevent overeruption. The resin can be easily removed when the bridge is fitted so restoring the desired occlusal contacts.

Clearly, these bridges should be completed as quickly as possible, because movement of teeth can always occur, particularly where there has been orthodontic treatment or where there is loss of bone from previous periodontal disease. Furthermore, in places where occlusal clearance has been created, space can quickly be lost by tooth movements.

The pontic space may be maintained with either a well-fitting and stable acrylic partial denture or a resin-bonded acrylic bridge using the method of Deubert and Jenkins (1982) who advocated that the pontic—a stock acrylic denture tooth—should have three essential design features to enhance the bonding to tooth (Box G).

The temporary resin-bonded bridge is quite easily removed with any of the methods described later. The remnants of the bonding resin adhering to the tooth surfaces may be polished down to the original level. Fresh resin may bond quite reliably to old, provided the latter has not been grossly contaminated.

Try-in procedure

With the proviso that the tooth surfaces have been isolated and cleaned with oil-free pumice, but have not been etched, the bridge may be carefully inserted in order to recognize the path of insertion, to check the fit and, to a lesser extent, to check the aesthetics and occlusion. The 'shine-through' effect also needs to be observed carefully—this is, the greyness of translucent enamel which is caused by the shadow of the metal flange. A test application of the luting resin can be made by merely applying the base component and observing its effect. Most of the current resins which are made specifically for resin-bonded bridges now contain opaquers and the problem of 'shine-through' is not so serious. If incisal greying cannot be obliterated even with opaque resins, then the flange may need to be cut well away from the incisal edge. If sufficient retention and a well-defined path of insertion are present, this reduction in the lingual bonding surface area will not be missed.

The etch metal bridges are especially sensitive to contamination from saliva, oil and dirt, which

BOX G ACRYLIC TEMPORARY BRIDGE

1 A slightly overlarge acrylic tooth should be selected and the approximal surfaces trimmed so that the pontic overlaps on the labial/buccal and lingual aspects of the abutment teeth (Figure 6.4). This creates a simple but effective means of providing a single path of insertion, thus ensuring correct location and stability of the pontic and so reducing the chances of bonding failure. Even if the bond fails, the pontic is less likely to be displaced and lost.
2 The pontic should fit closely to the abutment surfaces to keep the bonding resin as thin as possible.
3 Undercut channels should be prepared in the approximal surfaces of the pontic to provide mechanical retention for the bonding resin because the latter does not bond well to acrylic resin. Preferably, a composite resin should be used and, as a precaution, the approximal surfaces of the acrylic pontic should be primed with acrylic monomer before applying the composite resin bonding agent.

can easily clog up the minute pores on the etched surface, and preferably the trial fit should be carried out before metal etching has been done. Certainly, if a characterization of porcelain is necessary, this should be done and the restoration completely finished before metal etching is performed. Once the metal surfaces have been etched, no adjustments to the bridge should be made.

As mentioned in Chapter 2, the only reliable method of confirming that a casting has been etched is to use a laboratory microscope. Nevertheless, at the chairside the so-called 'water retention test' (Simonsen et al, 1983) can be employed to give an approximate indication of an etched metal surface (Figure 6.5). A drop of distilled water is placed on the flange, whereupon it will be drawn into the etched surface causing the latter to darken slightly. If a stream of air is then directed gently across the surface, the colour will slowly lighten as the water evaporates. A poorly etched or unetched surface will not display this effect and water would be blown readily off from the surface.

Bridges with cast-in mechanical retention, such as the mesh or particle-roughened types, pose less of a problem with try-ins. Nevertheless, these bridges cannot be temporarily cemented and therefore the patient must accept the aesthetic look before the bridge is finally cemented in place.

If there is a danger of contamination during try-in (bearing in mind that try-in for aesthetics may frequently have to take place without a rubber dam), the etched metal surface may be protected by painting on some unfilled bonding resin—this will flow into the pores to present an impervious film. This resin film should not be cured. Any saliva smearing the surface may be washed away easily and, when the bridge is cemented in place after cleaning, the resin film will bond readily to the luting resin.

All tried-in bridges should be cleaned in an ultrasonic cleaner with a proprietary cleaning agent before cementation. An effective course, especially where there has been gross contamination with saliva, is based on the work of Aboush and Jenkins (1987), as follows:

1 Rinse the bridge with running water from the tap.
2 Immerse in a beaker of detergent solution, eg Micro (International Products Corp.) pre-heated to 60°C.
3 Place the beaker in an ultrasonic bath and turn on the unit for 1–3 minutes.
4 Remove bridge and rinse with distilled water before drying with hot air.

Bridges treated with the Silicoater process pose a different problem. The SiO_x–C layer is relatively unstable and, once coated, the appliance can be stored for only 24 hours. If the coated surface is inadvertently contaminated, it has to be burnt off and the whole silanization process repeated. For this reason, it is recommended that the surface be protected with a thin layer of light-cured opaque resin.

Moisture control

Bonding techniques demand a fastidious approach to moisture control. The rubber dam is ideal in this respect, and is quickly and easily applied once the technique has been learnt. This is achieved not only from reading the several useful texts available (Elderton, 1971; Lynch and Tay, 1989), but more importantly by seeking the guidance of an experienced colleague or attending a 'hands-on' course at a postgraduate centre. Briefly, there are several important points regarding successful rubber dam application:

1. Purchase the right equipment. Pre-packed starter or basic kits are available from firms such as Ash Instruments and The Hygienic Corporation, but customized kits may be made up according to personal preferences from items bought separately. Medium to heavy grade rubber is best for bonding procedures.
2 The rubber dam technique is essentially a 'four-handed' procedure, and the collaboration of a trained chairside assistant saves much time and effort.
3 Thorough mechanical cleansing of the tooth, including the removal of calculus, is important before applying the rubber dam.
4 Isolate as many teeth as possible which are additional to those being etched—the more teeth that are isolated, the more securely is the rubber dam held in place, and the greater the access and visibility to the field of operation (Figure 6.6).

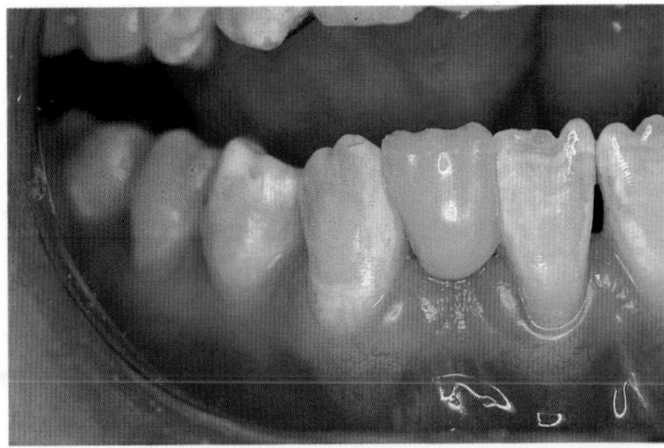

Figure 6.4

Temporary resin-bonded bridge made in acrylic resin to replace missing lower right lateral incisor. (a) Labial view;

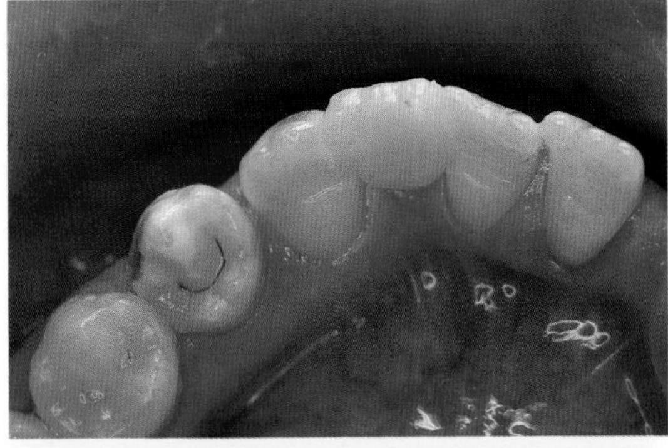

(b) incisal view showing close fit of the acrylic pontic which slightly overlaps the approximal surfaces of the abutment teeth.

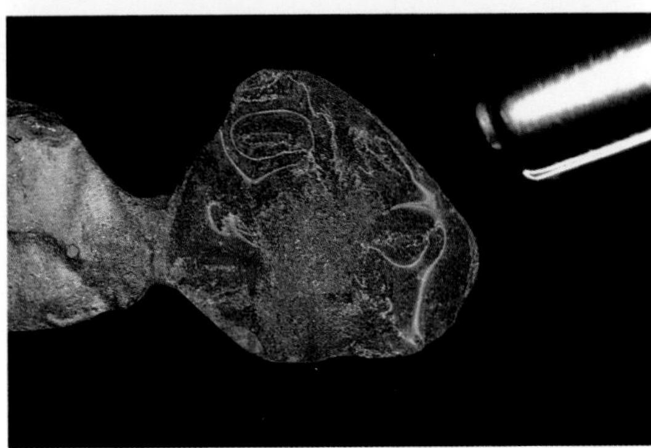

Figure 6.5

The 'water retention test' gives an approximate indication as to whether or not a metal surface has been adequately etched. (a) A drop of distilled water is placed on the etched surface causing it to darken slightly.

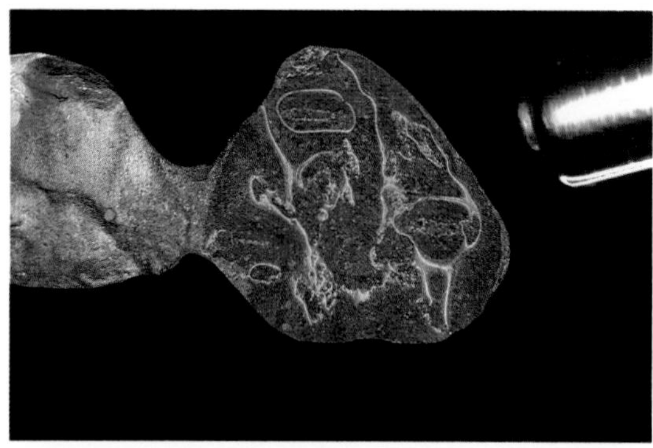

(b) A stream of air gently directed across the surface will gradually evaporate the film of water causing the metal to lighten again.

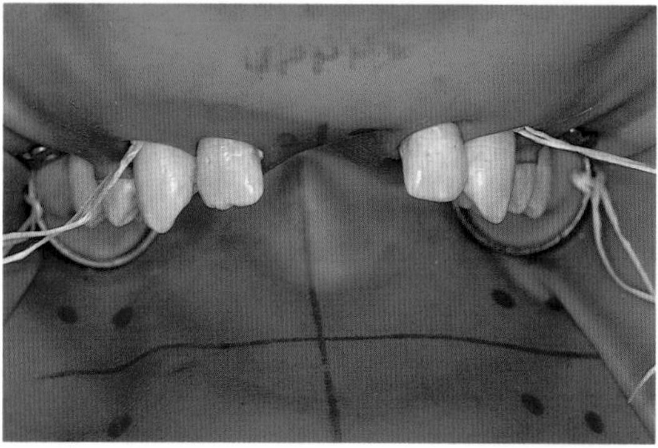

Figure 6.6

The complete isolation of teeth from moisture will enhance the success of etching procedures. The rubber dam is the ideal vehicle for this. (a) Labial view;

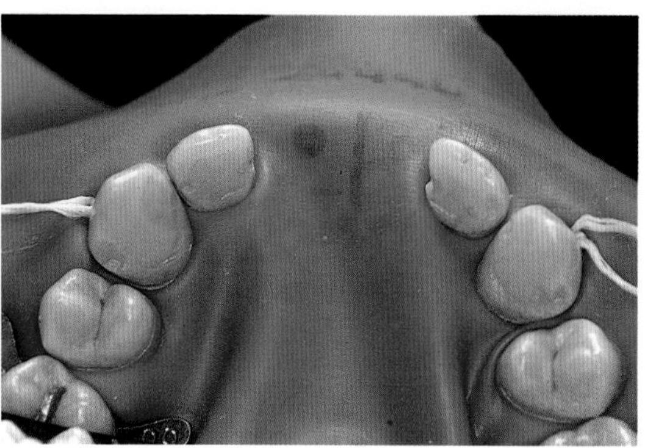

(b) palatal view. Note the number of teeth isolated by the rubber dam giving full access and visibility to the field of operation.

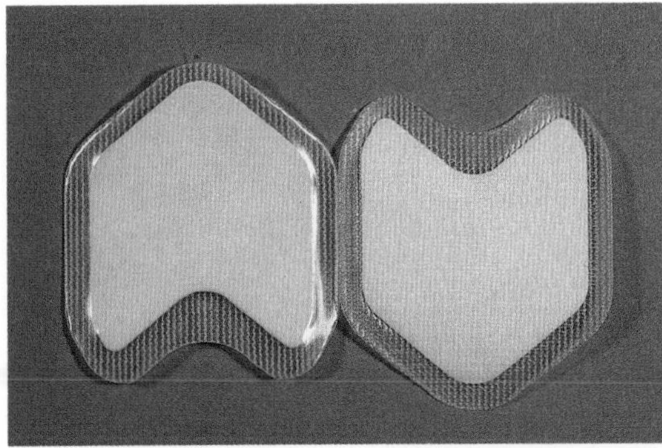

Figure 6.7

Dry Tips (Scandent) are a useful alternative in situations where a rubber dam is not feasible. (a) The Dry Tips wafers;

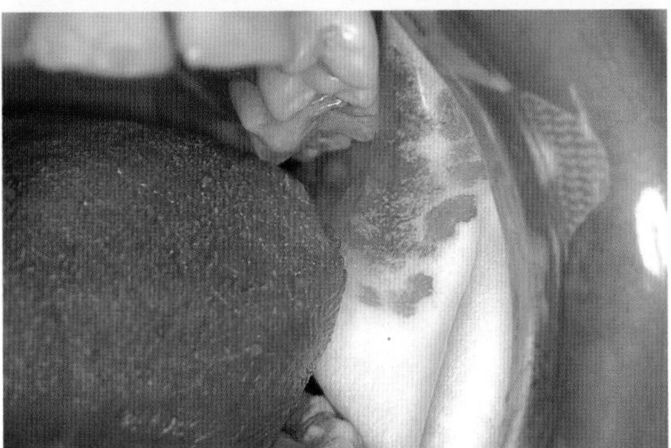

(b) the wafers in place over the parotid duct. The dark patches indicate the saturation with moisture.

5 Do not punch large holes in the rubber without due regard to the actual sizes of teeth being isolated. Although large holes make it easier to slip the rubber over a tooth, the loose fit at the neck of the tooth makes it difficult to evert the rubber cuff around the gingival crevice—essential if seepage of saliva is to be prevented.
6 Correct choice of clamps is also important.

Generally, for bonding purposes 'bland' clamps, ie those with jaws horizontally aligned (flat), are best for the purpose because they are gentle to the gingival tissues. They should grip the tooth all round, compressing the gingival tissues slightly. Care must be taken not to spill the phosphoric acid etchant on the clamps, particularly those made of martensitic carbon steel, which may suffer stress corrosion cracks when in contact with the acid even for a short time (Jedynakiewicz et al, 1985).

However, there may be occasions when it is not feasible to apply a rubber dam. Then, adequate isolation may be achieved by high-vacuum aspiration and cotton rolls. A particularly effective adjunct is a commercial nylon 'swab' called Dry Tips (Scandent) which contains a highly absorbent material—carboxymethylcellulose (Brady, 1986). This 'swab' is placed over the opening of the parotid duct and is very efficient in the volume of saliva it can absorb (Figure 6.7).

Etching the teeth

Although deceptively simple, acid etching of the teeth is a meticulous affair and each stage must be carried out scrupulously (Figure 6.8). Clinical success depends on understanding not only the outcome of each stage, but also the consequences of accidental or deliberate departure from the routine.

Step 1: Prophylaxis

As mentioned above, thorough cleaning or prophylaxis of the teeth to be etched should be carried out before applying the rubber dam. It is said that flavouring oils, glycerine and fluoride contained in the various commercial prophylaxis pastes may interfere with the quality of etch. However, so far no clinical or laboratory evidence has been offered to preclude the use of commercial pastes, even those containing fluoride.

Using a rubber polishing cup may be preferable to a bristle brush; the latter carries the risk of causing damage to the gingival tissues if it is clumsily applied and this, in turn, causes unnecessary bleeding and consequent contamination of the enamel surface. Both the bristle brush and the rubber cup are equally efficacious in removing plaque. After thorough prophylaxis, all remnants of polishing paste must be removed with copious washing.

Step 2: Isolation

The rubber dam is the most efficient and effective method of isolation of the teeth from saliva. This isolation step is often considered to be the most critical for successful acid-etch and bonding techniques.

Step 3: Etching

The etchant may be applied with a small bore syringe, fine brush (Figure 6.8a,b) or mini-sponge held in a pair of locking tweezers. The syringe and brush give greatest control over the area to be covered with the etchant. Gentle agitation and constant replenishment of the etchant should be adopted. Rubbing the enamel surface should be avoided because this burnishes the friable prisms and obliterates the etch pattern.

Step 4: Washing

Thorough washing with water from the dental syringe for at least 20 seconds removes unreacted phosphoric acid and the precipitates produced during etching (Figure 6.8c). Longer washing times, up to 60 seconds, may be required for etching gels in order to remove all trace of the viscous gel which becomes entrapped in the enamel micropores as a contaminant.

Step 5: Drying and re-isolation

After washing, the teeth should be dried immediately in a stream of warm air. Wet cotton rolls and absorbent swabs, if used instead of a rubber dam, should be changed. Although the dental air syringe is the most convenient to use, it should be checked periodically by blowing on a glass surface or a piece of blotting paper to ensure no water or oil is ejected with the air stream (Figure 6.9). Poorly maintained three-in-one syringes are particularly notorious for spurting out contaminants, and in such instances a miniature hairdrier may be used instead with maximum effect (Figure 6.8d,e). Commercial warm-air-driers, adapted specially for the acid-etch technique, are now available (Figure 6.10).

If the etching is successful, the surfaces should appear as a whitish matt with a 'lightly frosted' texture (Figure 6.8f). The resin should be applied immediately, because saliva or moisture contamination of freshly etched enamel for more than 1 second results in an adherent coating which cannot be removed successfully by washing (Silverstone et al, 1985). If saliva does contaminate the tooth surface before the resin can be applied, re-etching of the surface for 10 seconds will re-establish the etch pattern.

Insertion of bridge

Whatever the choice of resin, both operator and assistant must be familiar with the manufacturer's instructions. It is surprising how many mishaps occur through lack of care in the mixing and handling of the cement.

Small bridges may be easily loaded with the resin using the same mixing spatula, but with long-

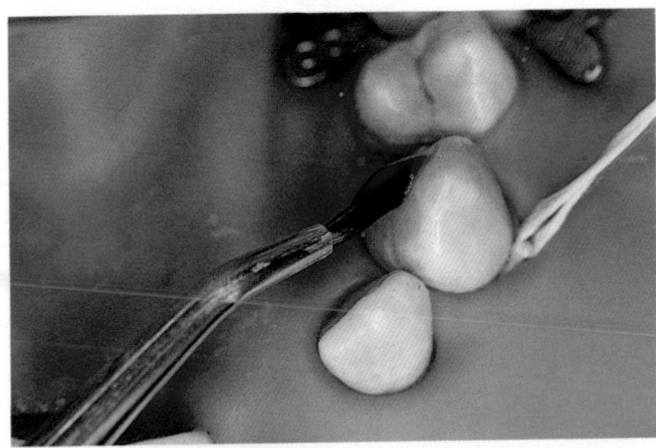

Figure 6.8

Etching procedure using a 37% phosphoric acid gel. (a) Application of the gel with a fine brush.

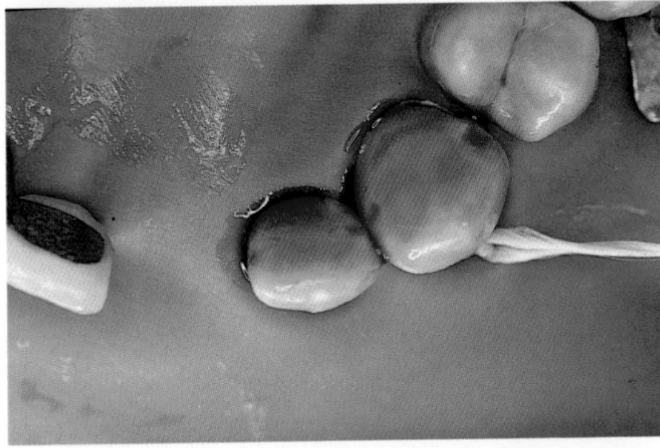

(b) Gel in place—almost all commercial gels are coloured to make them conspicuous against the tooth surface.

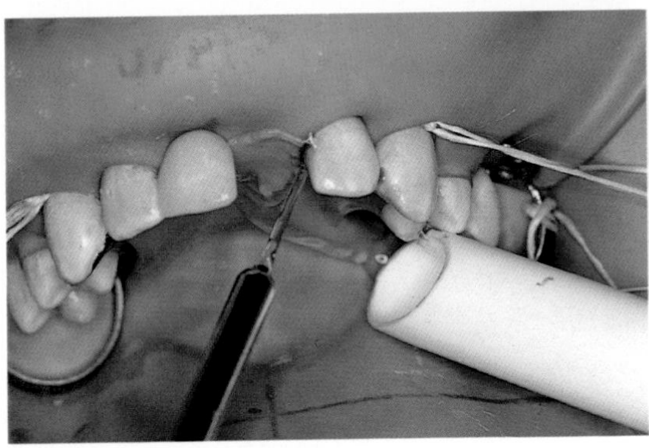

(c) Rinsing off the gel with a jet of water.

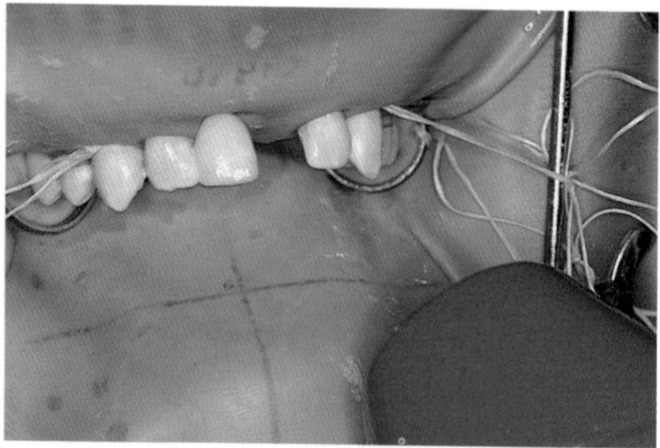

(d, e) Drying the tooth surfaces with a domestic hair-drier.

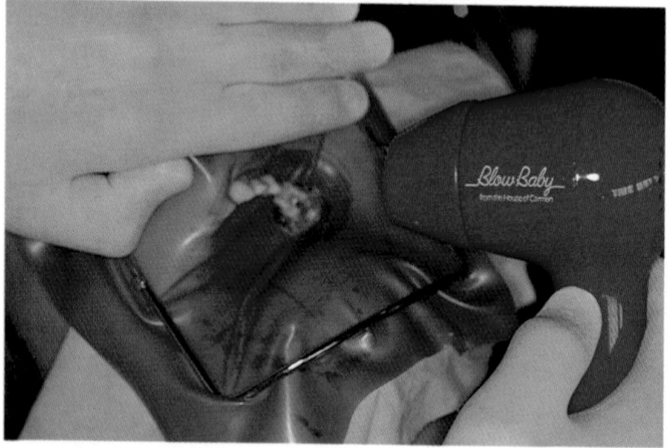

Note the placement of the gloved hand over the patient's face to shield the eyes and nose from the hot air.

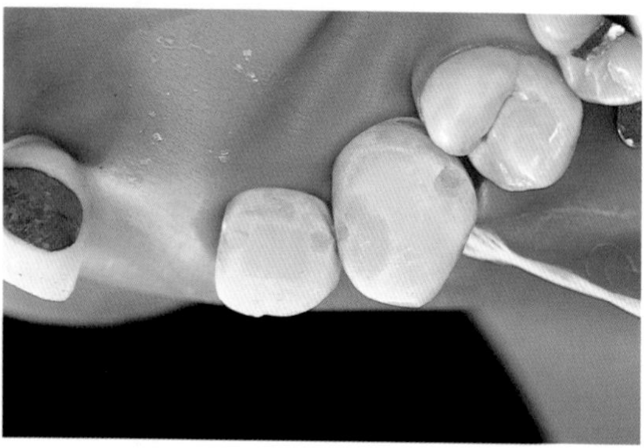

(f) A thoroughly dry, etched tooth surface shows the characteristic 'frosted' appearance.

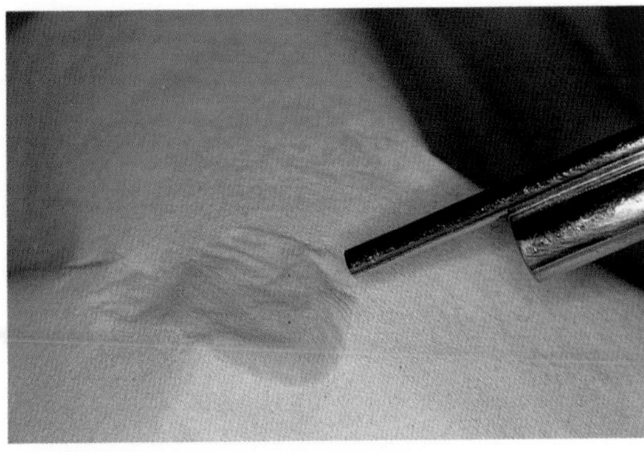

Figure 6.9

Testing a three-in-one syringe: a moist patch appearing on the paper towel while the 'air' button only is depressed indicates a leak in the system.

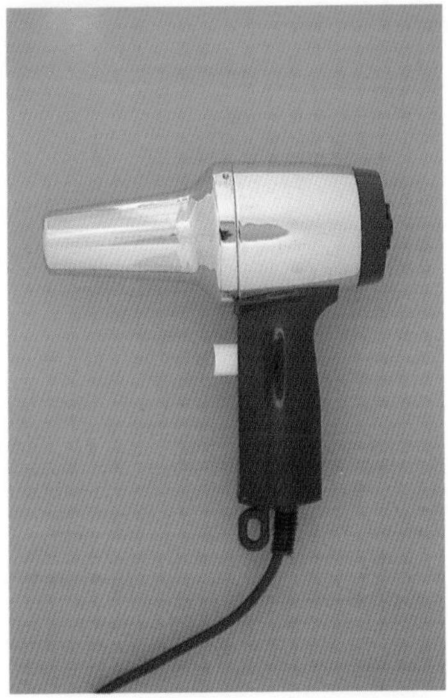

Figure 6.10

(a) The Handidry (Den-Mat Corp.) custom made for dental applications;

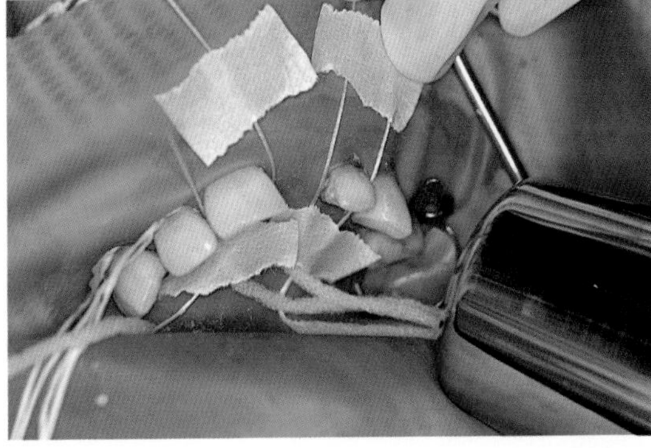

(b) the Handidry in action.

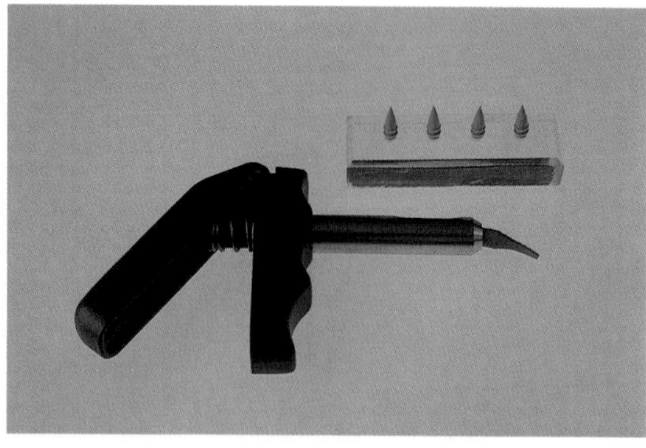

Figure 6.11

(a) The C-R Syringe (Centrix Incorporated);

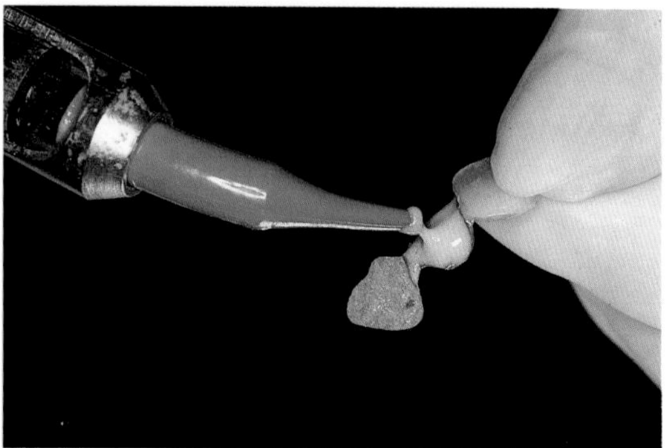

(b) a void-free layer of cement may be deposited on the metal with the syringe.

span bridges bearing several flanges, use of a syringe, such as the C-R Syringe (Centrix Incorporated), may be more convenient (Figure 6.11). The injection technique also lessens the chances of air bubbles forming in the resin layer.

A few simple precautions, taken to prevent excess resin from clogging the embrasures, will save the later embarrassment and frustration of trying to remove the set resin with burs, and subsequently trying to polish a framework roughened by such removal.

Before the bridge is cemented in place, the dental assistant holds the leader thread of a length of Super Floss (Oral B) against the abutment teeth. If a rubber dam is in place the Super Floss itself may be taped in position temporarily with short lengths of a low adhesive drafting tape (3M Co.) while the assistant mixes the cement (Figure 6.12a). Then, with the operator holding the bridge in place, the tapes are removed and the assistant passes the floss through the embrasures several times to clean the area of excess resin (Figure 6.12b–d). A small paint brush or dental explorer may also be used for this purpose. Self-adhesive, thin metal or plastic foils or strips (Hawe-Neos Dental), or very soft mouldable metal strips (eg Dead-Soft Metal Strip, Den-Mat Corp.), which have been adapted to the tooth surfaces distal to the abutment teeth, may help to prevent seepage of the resin into the contact areas (Figure 6.12c). Incidentally, these metal strips may also serve as protective barriers to accidental spread of acid during the etching procedures.

If a single path of insertion has been incorporated in the design by appropriate tooth preparations, there should be no difficulty in locating the bridge accurately. A template or index may be made from a silicone impression putty to confirm and assist in accurate seating (Figure 6.13). Often,

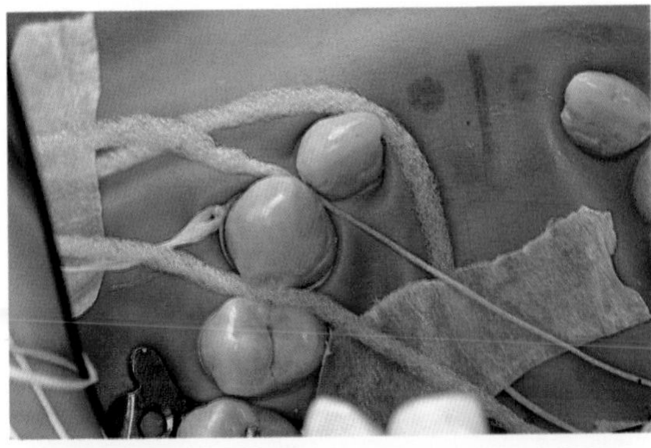

Figure 6.12

(a) Super Floss (Oral B) passed approximally between the abutment teeth. The free ends of the floss are taped to the rubber dam.

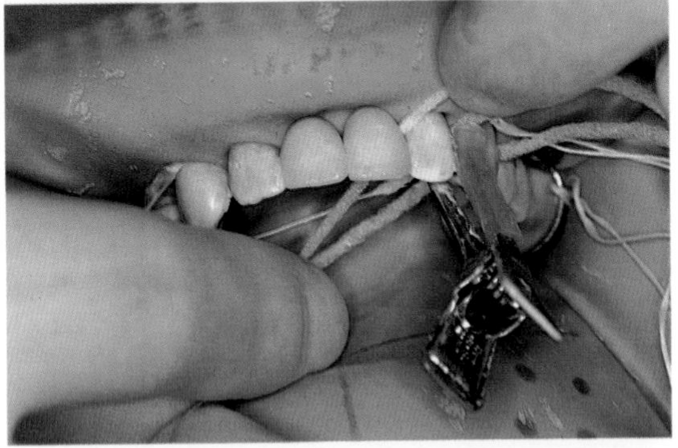

(b) After inserting the bridge, the tapes are peeled off and the floss passed through the embrasures to remove excess cement.

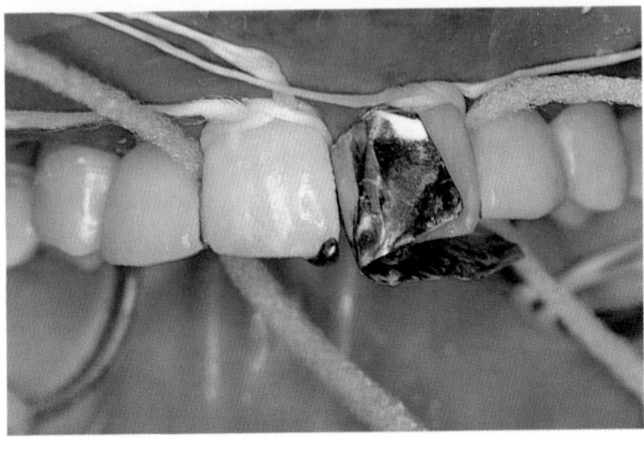

(c) Dead-Soft Metal Strips (Den-Mat Corp.) are also useful in preventing excess cement from clogging up the embrasures.

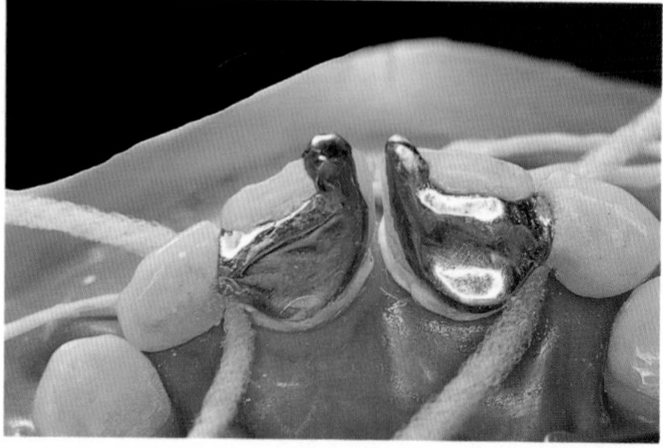

(d) Palatal view showing passage of Super Floss through the embrasures. The flanges of these two cantilever bridges have hooked extensions over the incisor edges of the central incisor teeth to lend additional support while the cement is setting.

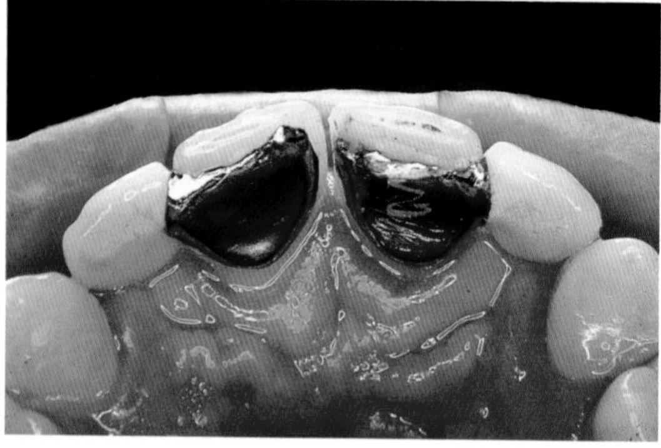

(e) After the cement has set the hooks are removed with a bur, and the cut area polished before the patient is dismissed.

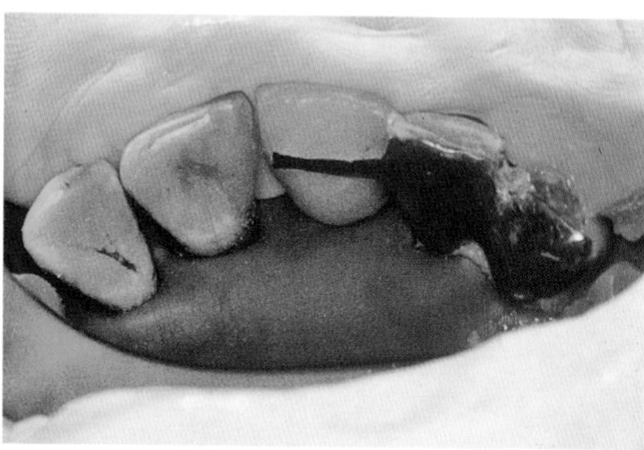

Figure 6.13

Location of cantilever bridges during cementation may also be achieved with a silicone putty index.

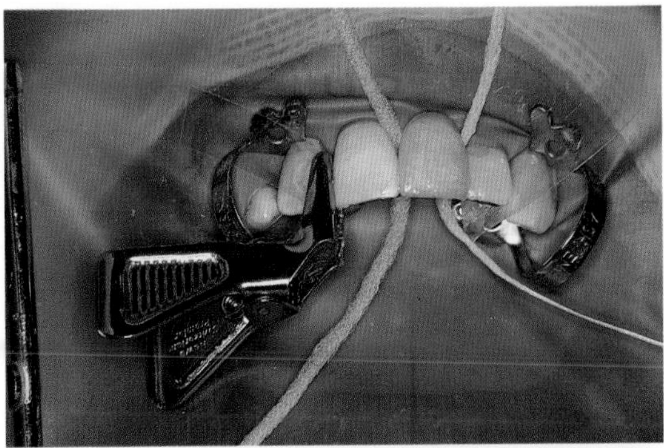

Figure 6.14

Suitably modified matrix strip clamps (Hawe-Neos) may be useful in holding the bridge in place during cementation. (a) Labial view;

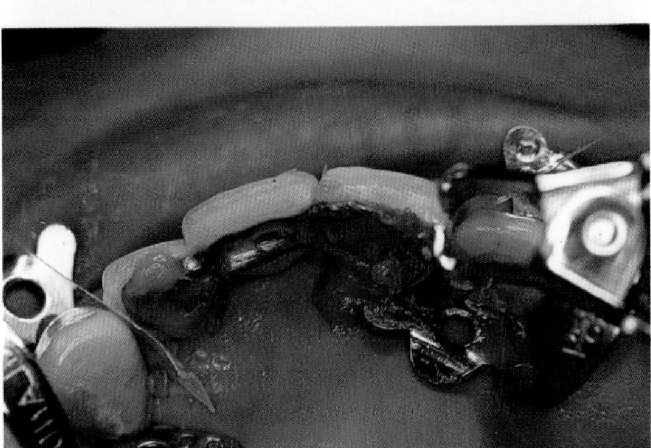

(b) palatal view. Blue Panavia-EX Oxyguard (Kuraray) covers the flanges.

small support hooks, which extend from the flange over the incisal edges or cusp tips, may help to locate and hold the bridge steady during the setting of the resin (Figure 6.12d). These hooks are later cut off with a bur (Figure 6.12e). Such seating aids are particularly useful for cantilever bridges, but not essential for successful cementation, and it is more important to achieve a 'positive' fit in the first instance.

The bridge is held in place with finger pressure, but suitably adapted strip-clamps (Hawe-Neos Dental Nos 111 and 111A) may be used as convenient 'stabilizers' for anterior bridges (Figure 6.14). The jaws of these clamps have sharp serrated teeth which must be filed or ground down and sleeved with polythene tubing (Figure 6.15). They are most effective in the lower incisor region where the slopes of the marginal ridges of the abutment teeth are almost vertical (Figure 6.16).

Any remaining excess of the set resin is removed with sharp scalers and the margins of the flanges are finished with micro-diamond stones and 30-bladed tungsten carbide finishing burs, followed by white composite finishing stones. Finishing should be carried out in a dry field to help detect excess resin, and the direction of rotation of the burs should preferably be from metal to tooth. If necessary, final polish is achieved by light buffing with bonded abrasive points. Use of heavy pressure during polishing should be avoided. The amount of heat generated may soften the underlying resin and jeopardize the bond.

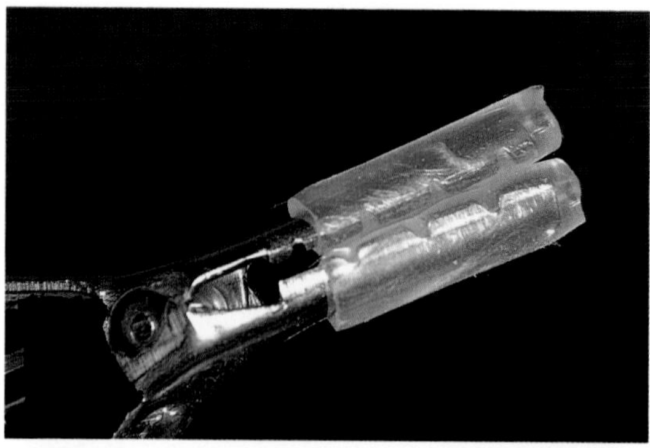

Figure 6.15

The sharp, serrated jaws of the matrix strip clamp are ground flat and sleeved with polythene tubing.

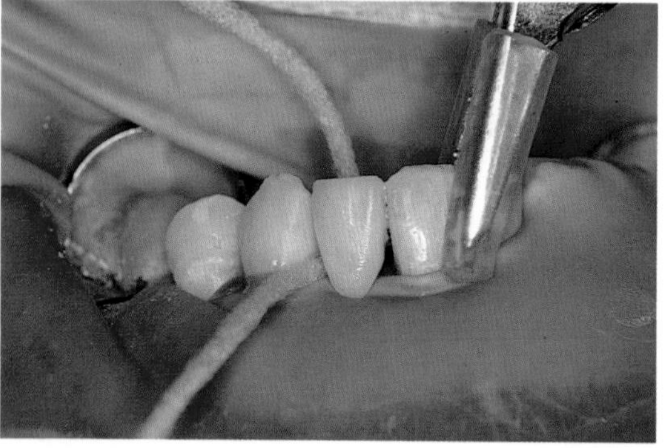

a

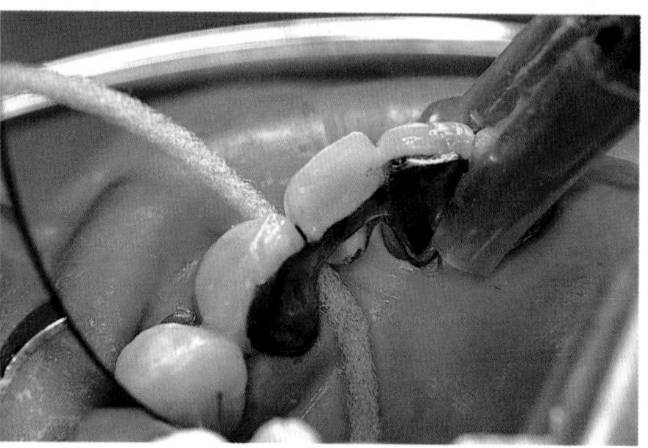

b

Figure 6.16 (a, b)

Modified matrix strip clamps retaining a bridge in position during cementation.

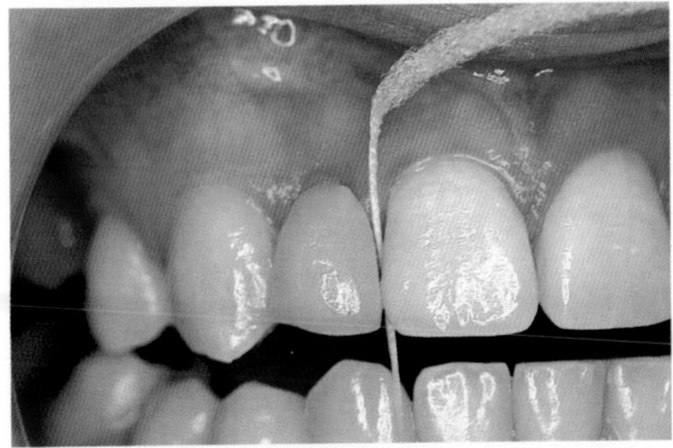

Figure 6.17

Cleaning of the bridge by the patient is important, and Super Floss is an ideal adjunct to regular toothbrushing. (a) The nylon filament assists in threading the floss through the embrasure;

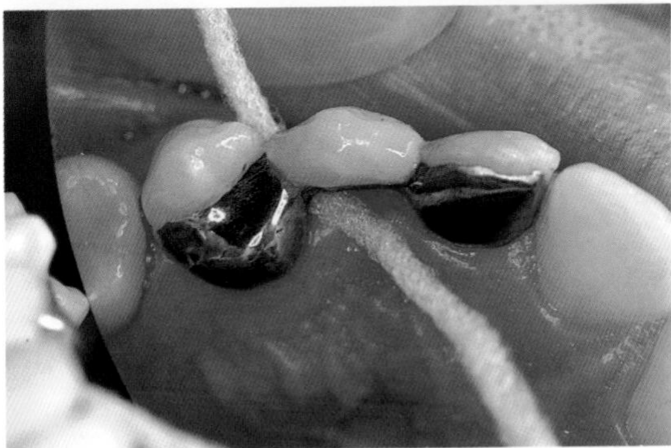

(b) palatal view. The floss must be passed under and around the pontic.

Final assessment of occlusion

Tooth contacts in the ICP should first be tested with plastic strips (shimstock) in the mouth, and then the same contacts should be verified on the mounted casts if these are available. Other materials which may be used are the various proprietary occlusal indicator waxes and films. At this stage, only the most minor adjustments (if any) should be carried out. Again, excessive grinding and polishing of the metal flanges may generate too much heat and should be avoided.

Occlusal adjustments using guidance copings are accomplished at this stage. Again, the contacts should be tested and verified with shimstock. Ground occlusal surfaces should be smoothed with graded abrasive discs and coated with a fluoride varnish for further protection.

Final assessment of aesthetics

If all has gone well, the patient should be pleased with the result. At this stage it is difficult and, indeed, inadvisable to alter the shade or form of the pontic. However, if necessary, some minor tinting can be carried out with proprietary porcelain repair kits and a suitable tinted resin.

Oral hygiene instruction and home care

By now the patient should be aware of the importance of maintaining good oral hygiene and have received instructions on how to carry out the various procedures, such as using plaque disclosing

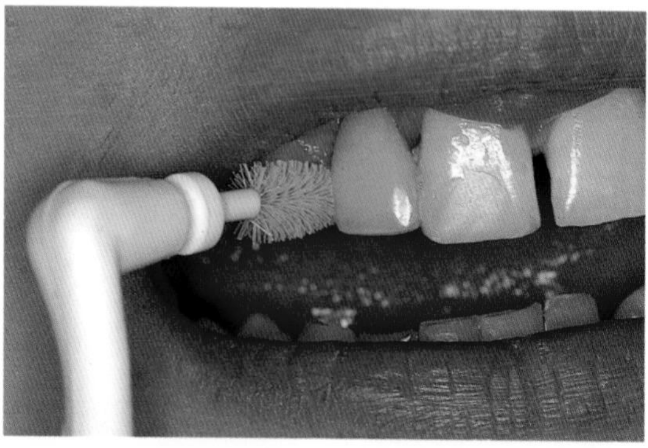

Figure 6.18

Small 'interproximal' brushes (eg Oral B) may be used to clean the bridge. (a) Brush being passed through an embrasure.

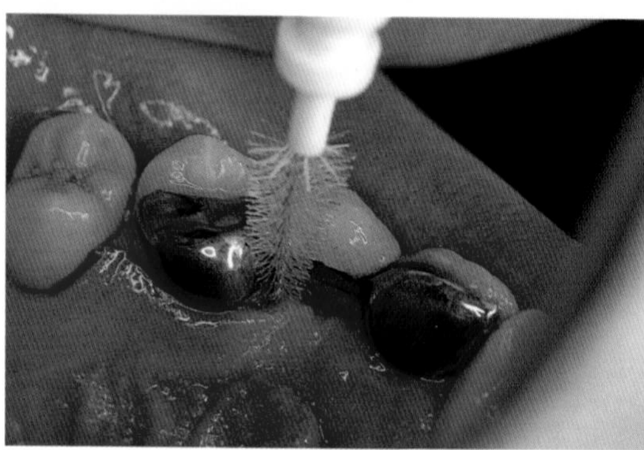

(b) View from the palatal side.

solutions, tooth brushing, interdental stimulators and dental floss.

Nevertheless, a special discipline is required both to care for a bridge and to ensure the supporting tissues do not suffer from neglect. There are two particular areas that need attention:

1 The embrasure and interdental area.
2 The mucosa under the pontic.

Super Floss (Oral B) is one of the most effective bridge-cleaning aids. It may be passed through the interdental area and underneath the pontic. There are three parts, namely a stiff filament to facilitate the insertion of a 'spongy' middle section which is particularly useful for cleaning underneath smooth saddle pontics. A length of regular floss thread, attached to the other end of the 'spongy' section, makes up the rest of the Super Floss (Figure 6.17).

Once it has been passed through the interdental space, the floss is held tightly and rubbed against the surfaces of the tooth and retainer. It may be negotiated underneath the pontic to keep the surface clean (Figure 6.17b). Other methods of removing plaque from the embrasure spaces are the small 'interdental' or 'interproximal' brushes (Figure 6.18), and there are several commercial kits available.

Finally, the patient is advised to take care to avoid sudden impact on the bridge, as might occur in chewing nuts. If the patient's leisure activities include contact sports or vigorous games, such as squash, then he or she would be well advised to consider wearing a mouthguard.

Accidental damage to crowns and bridges can

often be caused by anaesthetists and, if the patient is anticipating an operation under general anaesthesia, it would be sensible to warn the anaesthetist of the presence of the bridge.

Routine bridge checks

It is advisable to see the patient again within a fortnight, and subsequently at monthly intervals for the first 6 months. Most bonding and other failures tend to occur during this period, but the prognosis tends to improve as the months and years go by. Thus, after the initial 6 months, the patient may be recalled at 6-monthly intervals for the next 2 years and then just for an annual check-up thereafter.

The patient should be asked if he or she has experienced any discomfort or anything untoward with the bridge, assuming of course that he or she is satisfied with the appearance of the bridge: Is the occlusion correct? Does the bridge feel loose? Any problem of which the patient has become aware should be dealt with first, especially if pain or pulpal sensitivity is the prominent symptom.

The area around the bridge should be examined to see how efficiently the patient's oral hygiene routine has been performed. Where there are lapses, the patient should be reminded of the importance of keeping the bridge free of plaque. If necessary, the correct brushing and flossing procedures should be reiterated. Inflammation around and underneath the pontic may suggest poor oral hygiene or, more seriously, a loose, poorly supported bridge causing friction on the mucosa (Figures 6.19 and 6.20).

Mobility, pocketing and the bleeding index of the abutment teeth should be recorded and compared with the initial state. It is also useful to examine the corresponding teeth on the opposite side to ascertain whether periodontal breakdown is localized to the bridge or affects the whole mouth.

After this, the occlusion is checked noting carefully any undue movement of the bridge in lateral and protrusive excursions. Contacts may again be tested with shimstock. On the surfaces of the metal flanges, any shiny wear facets should be noted and confirmed with occlusal indicator waxes or coloured occlusal tape. Minor adjustment may be carried out if necessary.

The integrity of the flanges is now examined. If a Rochette bridge has been fitted, the amount of composite resin loss from the perforations should be noted. Partial bonding failure may be indicated in the following ways:

1 The patient tells you that the bridge feels loose.
2 With a large spoon excavator applied to the cervical margin of the flange, pull down firmly on each of the retainers and observe any movement. Use of a pair of magnifying loupes will greatly assist in the detection of minute discrepancies.
3 Press on each retainer in turn with a ball-ended burnisher. Bubbles forming in the fluid around the margins usually indicate a bond failure.

Caries

A danger with partial debonds is the onset of caries, and the same holds true for a leaky conventional bridge. In the case of resin-bonded bridges, the tell-tale signs are often a discoloration of the abutment tooth and underlying resin (Figure 6.21). It is important to investigate any complaint of 'looseness' before irreparable damage occurs.

Radiographs should be taken to confirm the presence, and establish the extent, of caries. Vitality tests may also be performed if there is any doubt about the state of the pulp. The management of bond failures is considered in the next section.

Finally, if all is well, the patient may be dismissed until the next recall appointment, but should be reminded of the importance of returning immediately if any mishap befalls the bridge.

The management of bond failures (debonds)

Debonds are probably the most common failure affecting resin-bonded bridges and may be classified as 'complete', ie with the bridge fully dislodged, or 'partial', where one or more flanges have detached but otherwise the bridge remains in place held by the remaining flange or flanges.

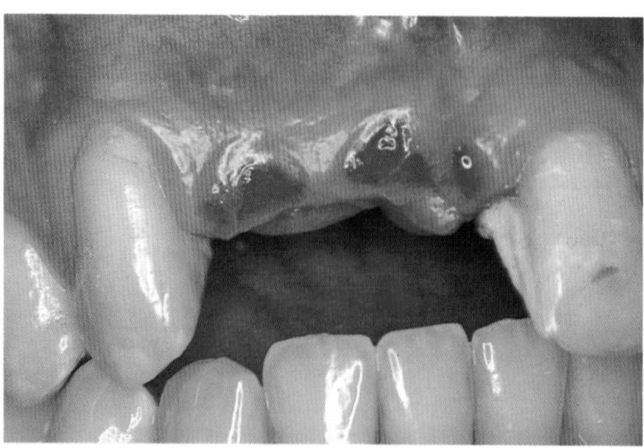

Figure 6.19

Friction on the mucosa caused by a loose and unhygienic bridge has resulted in severe inflammation.

Figure 6.20

(a) A badly designed bridge with minimal retention and support has impinged on the mucosa of the saddle area.

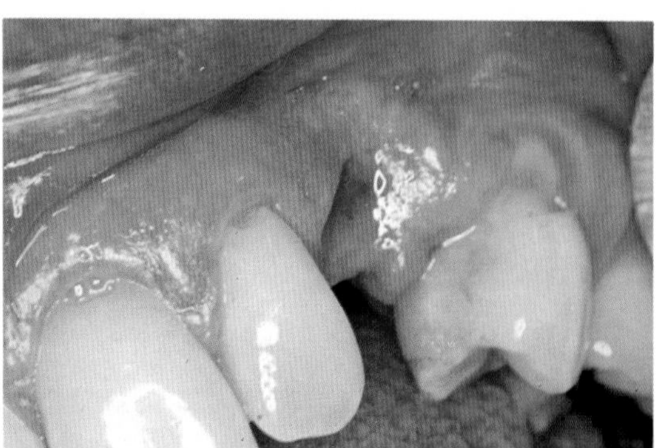

(b) This has resulted in inflammation and ulceration of tissue in contact with the pontic.

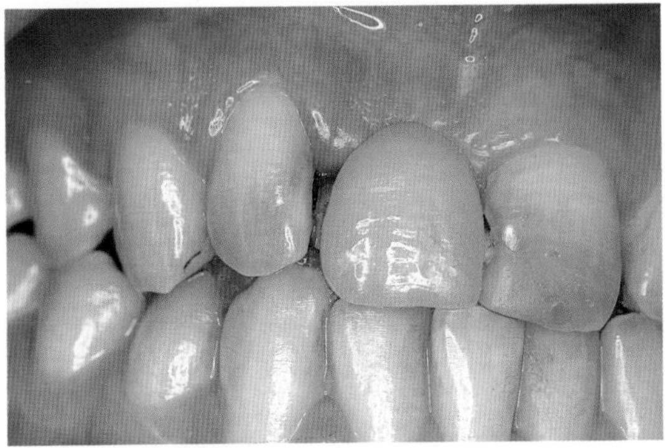

a

Figure 6.21

Often the first indication that caries has occurred under a resin-bonded bridge is discoloration of the affected tooth. (a) A bridge spanning the upper right canine to the upper left lateral incisor. Discoloration is present on both right lateral and central incisor abutment teeth, but caries is now fairly extensive as indicated by the radiograph in (b).

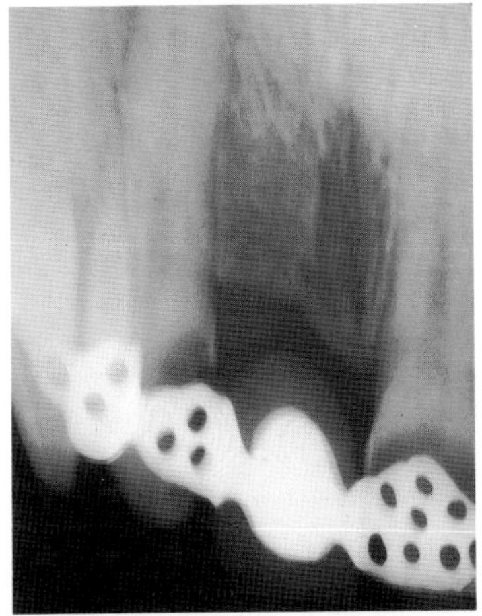

b

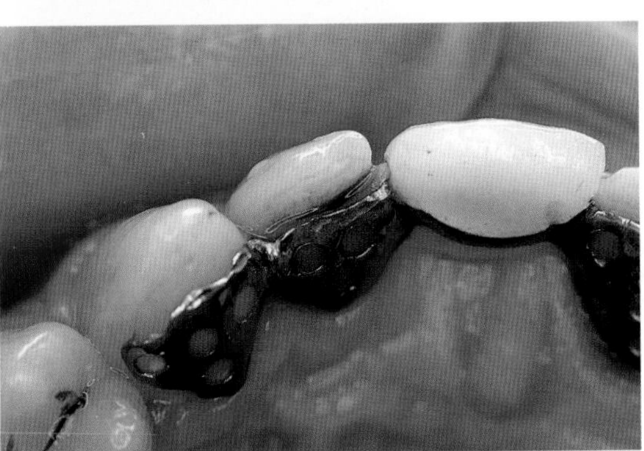

c

(c) Palatal view showing the loose flange, which when removed showed a deep carious lesion (d).

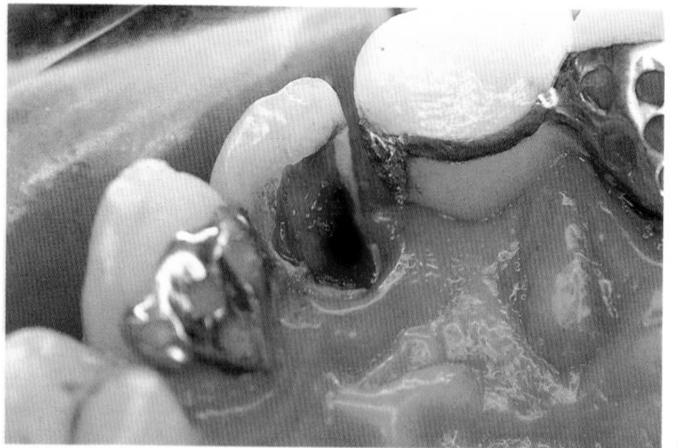

d

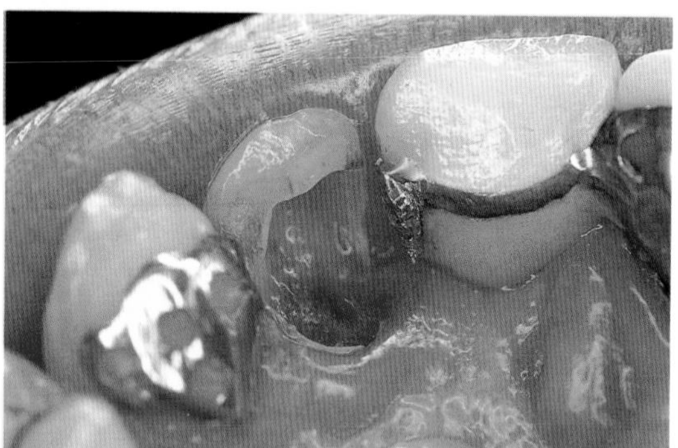

e

In (e), removal of caries reveals a near pulp exposure. Eventually, endodontic treatment was carried out on the abutment teeth and the old bridge replaced with a 'conventional' one.

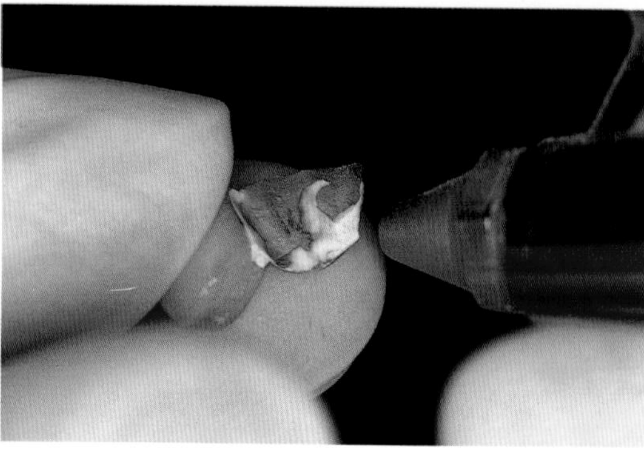

Figure 6.22

Cleaning the surface of metal by sandblasting with an airbrush.

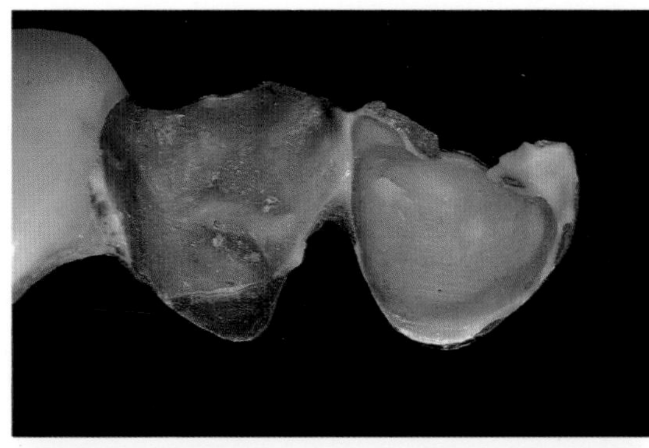

Figure 6.23
(a) Old and contaminated resin on the surface of metal flanges before burning off in a furnace.

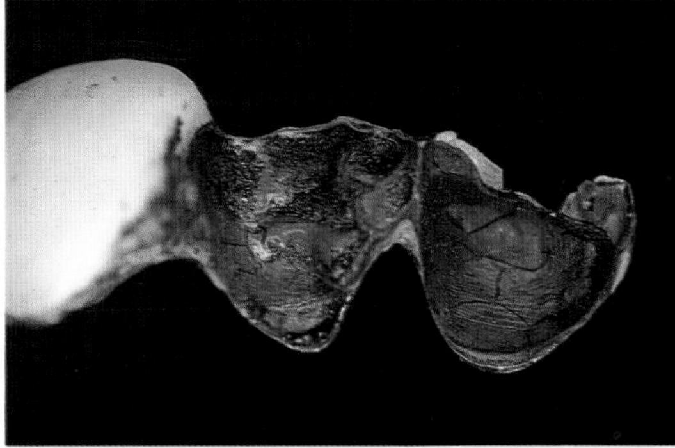

(b) Carbonization occurs if insufficiently high temperatures are used.

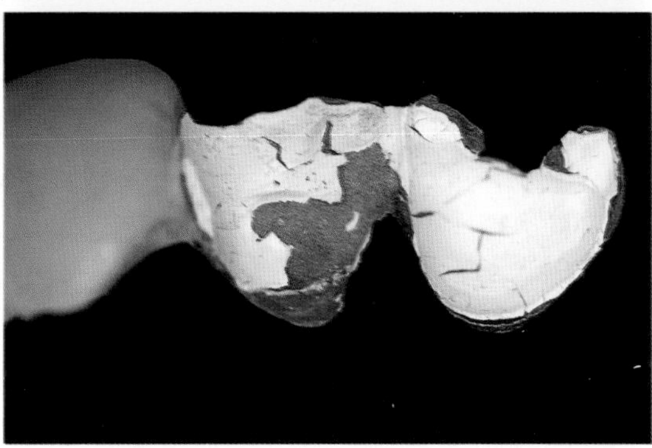

(c) At the correct temperature, the resin turns chalky white and then vaporizes.

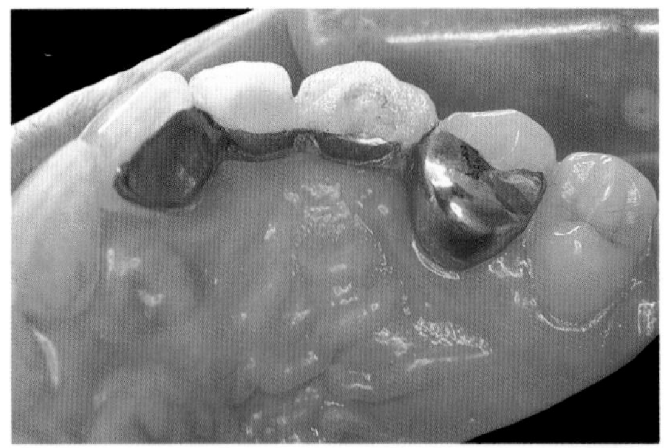
a

Figure 6.24

Fixed–fixed, resin-bonded bridge spanning upper left central incisor to upper left first premolar. (a) The flange on the central incisor has come adrift but the flange on the premolar is substantial and is holding the bridge in place.

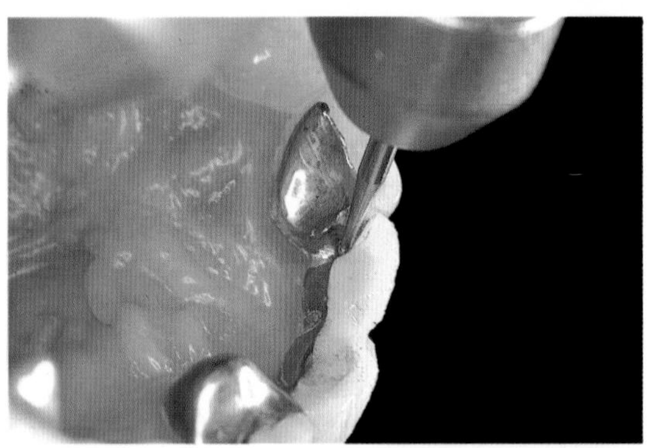
b

(b) The loose flange is removed with a round diamond bur, leaving the bridge supported only by the premolar as a cantilever design (c).

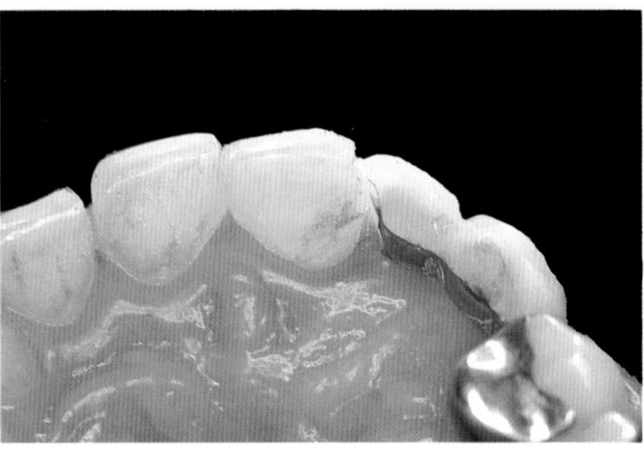
c

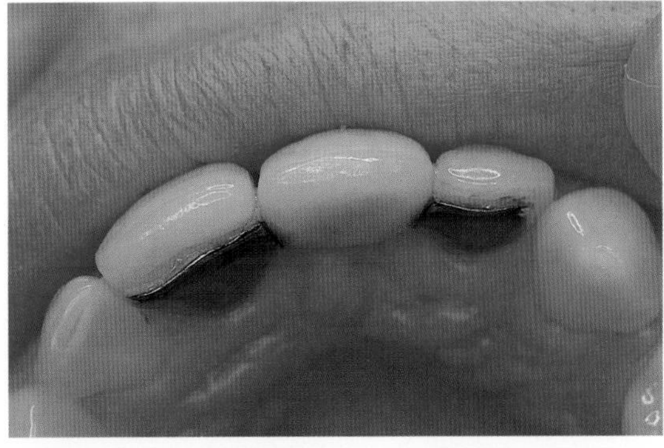

Figure 6.25

Resin-bonded bridge replacing upper left central incisor. (a) The flange on the left lateral incisor has loosened (debonded).

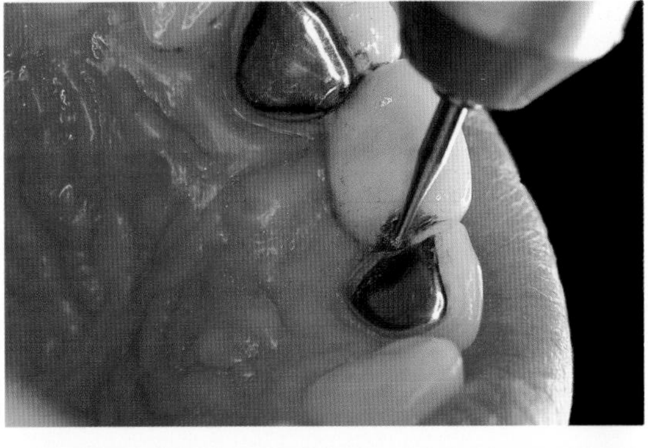

(b) The loose flange is removed with a round diamond bur.

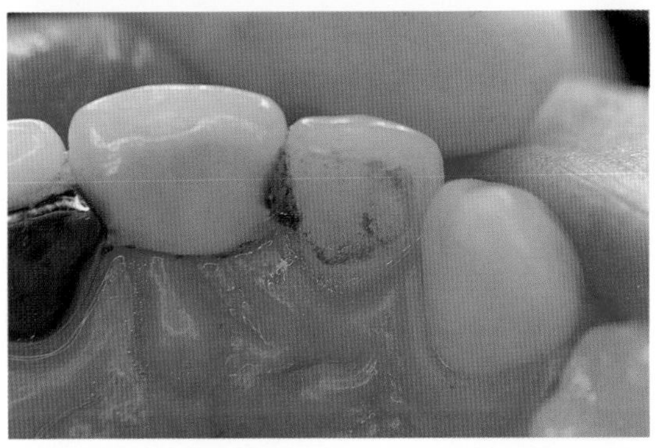

(c) There is a remnant of old stained resin on the tooth, but otherwise there is no evidence of caries.

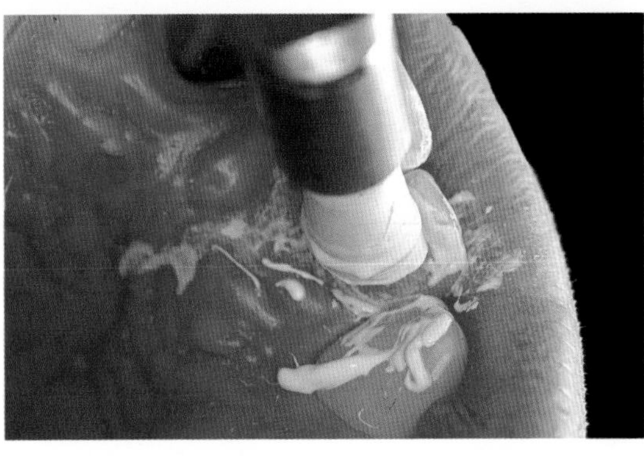

(d) The old resin was ground away and the tooth cleaned with a rubber cup and abrasive polish.

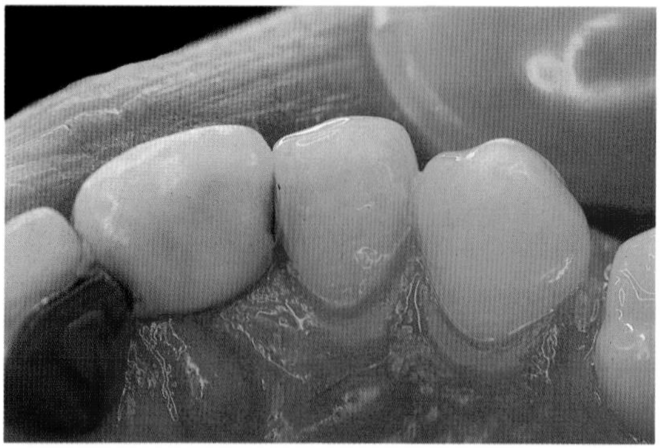

(e) The bridge is functioning well as a cantilevered design.

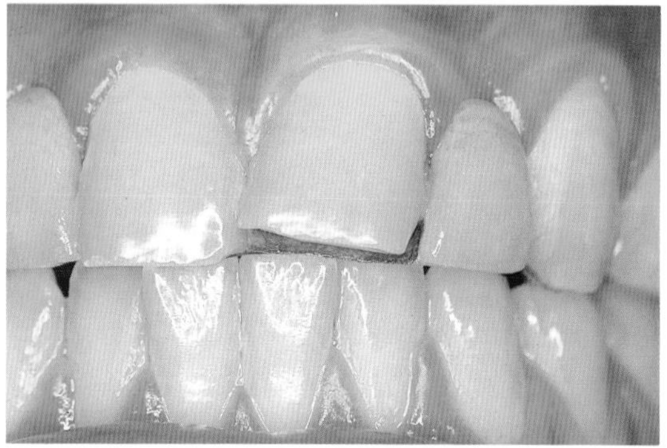

Figure 6.26

One-piece, six-unit, resin-bonded bridge replacing upper lateral incisors. (a) The upper left central incisor has become detached from the flange and is drifting labially under occlusal forces.

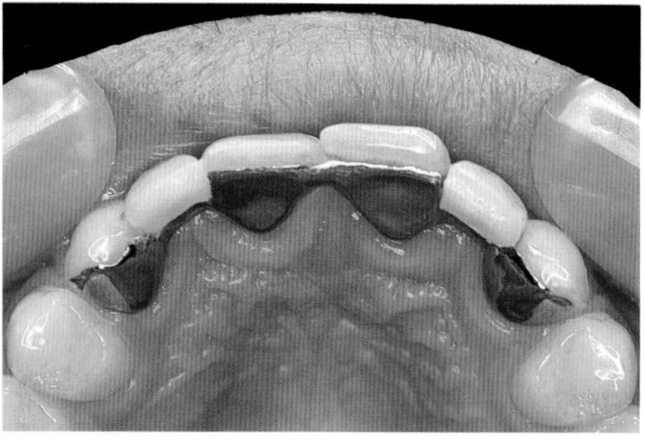

(b) Palatal view of the bridge. The splinting of the four abutment teeth is probably unnecessary and superfluous in terms of the narrow spans.

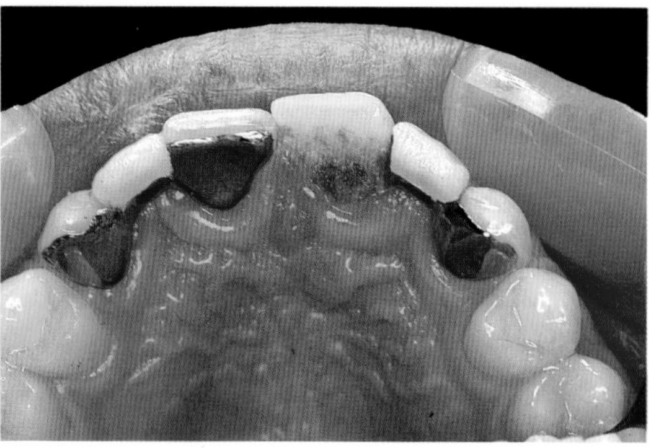

(c) The loose flange has been removed, showing staining and caries on the surface of the central incisor. The tooth was restored with a glass-ionomer cement. The bridge is functioning satisfactorily as a cantilevered unit.

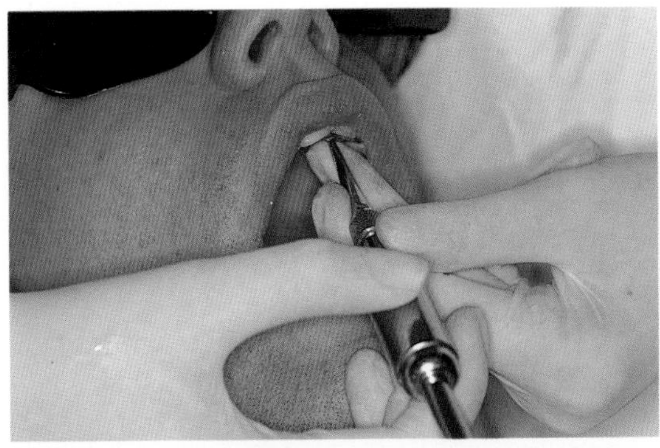

Figure 6.27

Falling-weight bridge remover in position.

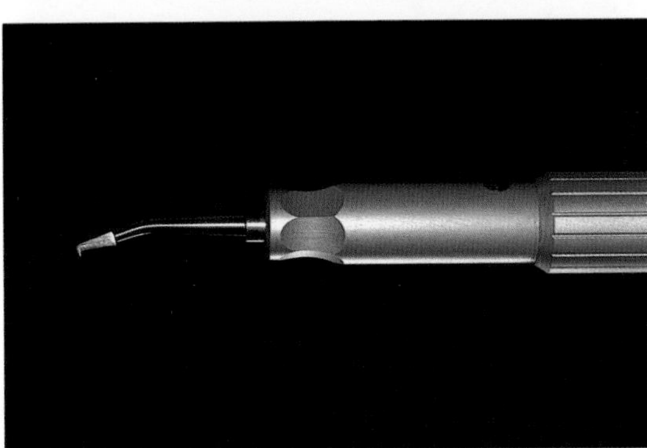

Figure 6.28

(a) The Automatic Crown Remover (Anthogyr S.A.) is a spring-loaded handpiece driven by a dental micromotor and delivers a preset vibratory force to the margins of the flanges.

The majority of debonds tend to occur at the metal–resin interface; sometimes the failure is between tooth and resin, and occasionally there is cohesive failure within the resin itself.

Complete debond

If the bridge is serviceable, it may be rebonded in place. All traces of adherent resin on the flange should be removed by sandblasting with aluminium oxide abrasive powder of 50–250 μm grit size in an airbrush (Figure 6.22). Alternatively, the resin may be burnt off in a porcelain furnace at 700°C for 10–15 minutes or longer (Simonsen et al, 1983). High temperatures are necessary to vaporize the resin completely and avoid the formation of excessive carbon deposits (Figure 6.23). This procedure is especially suitable for the etched-metal Maryland bridges, because it is said to reduce the chances of damaging the fragile etched patterns. A recent study has shown that burning off the resin does not affect the chances of a successful rebond (Haywood et al, 1990). Nevertheless, some practitioners may feel, in any case, that it is probably safer to re-etch the metal. Of course, the burn-out method is unsuitable if the pontic has been made of acrylic.

The metal flange may then be treated in one of the following ways:

1 With perforated, mesh, bead and other forms of mechanical retention, the bridge only needs to be cleaned in an ultrasonic machine before rebonding.

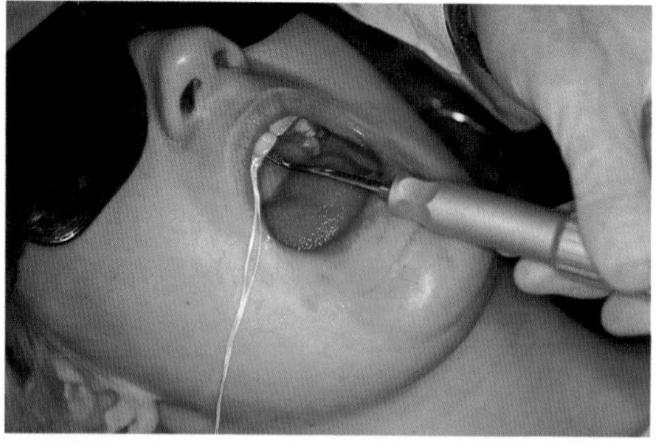

(b) Instrument in position: the operator's free hand should be supporting the bridge.

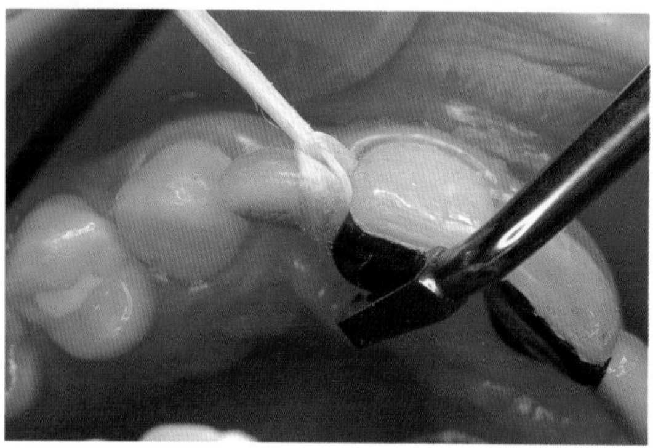

(c) Dental floss tape may be tied around the bridge to prevent it slipping accidentally down the throat. The free end of the tape may be looped around a button on the patient's clothing or held by the dental assistant.

2 With Maryland bridges, the bridge may be returned to the laboratory for re-etching, or etching may be carried out on the premises with chairside etching units or special hydrofluoric acid gels.
3 With nickel–chrome alloys, sandblasting alone with a 250-μm grit aluminium oxide abrasive powder may be all that is required and, when used with a so-called bifunctional resin such as Panavia EX high bond strengths of resin to metal can be expected.
4 Using the Inzoma method to lay on a porous metal coating as described in Chapter 2.
5 Tin-plating the sandblasted surface if the bridge has been made from gold alloys (see Chapter 2).
6 If no sandblasting or etching facilities are available, the quickest solution is to convert the bridge to a Rochette design by drilling holes in the flanges. Although this may seem a wasteful and desperate measure, in some circumstances it may prove to be as effective as any of the previous methods described.

Partial debond

Detachment of a single flange at either end of the bridge should not require the complete removal of the bridge in every case. Provided the remaining flange(s) is judged to be securely retained and that occlusal problems were not the initial cause of the debond, it would be feasible simply to remove the loose flange and leave the rest of the bridge in situ as a cantilever bridge (Tay, 1987). A

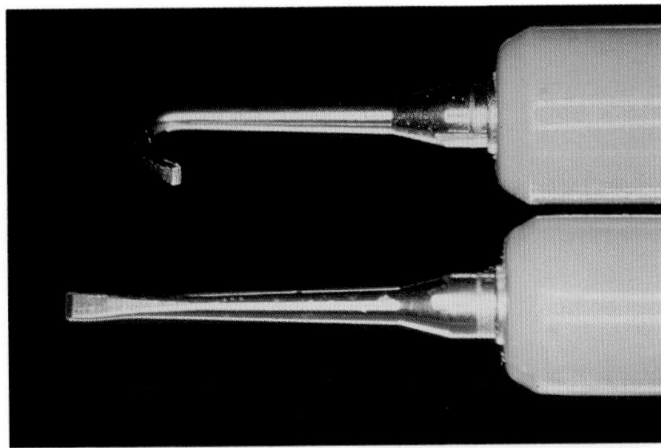

Figure 6.29

(a) The KJ Cavitron Inserts (De Trey/Dentsply) showing curved and straight points.

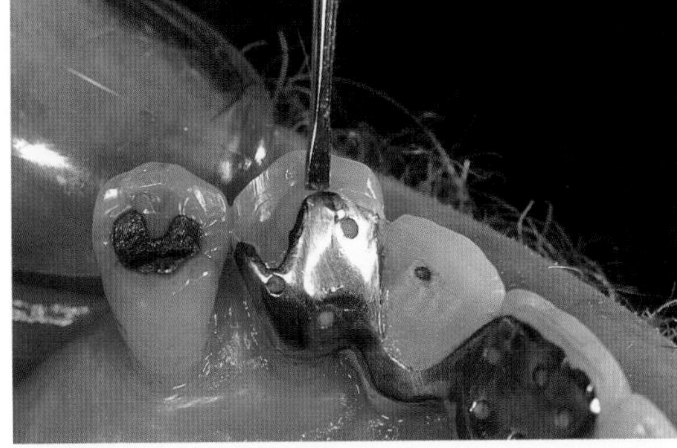

(b) Straight point applied to occlusal margin of flange.

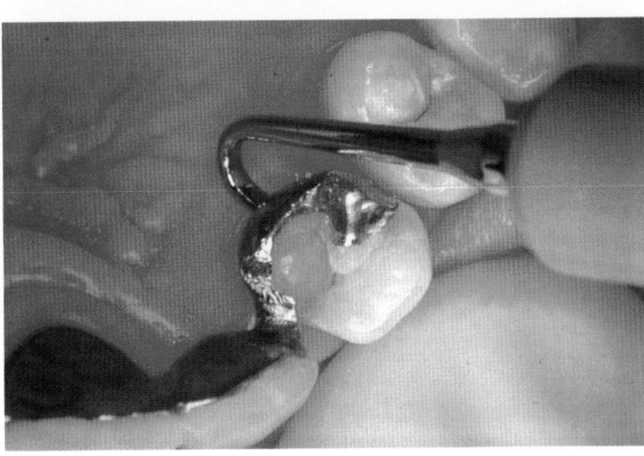

(c) Curved point applied to gingival margin of flange.

small, round, diamond bur may be used for this purpose (Figures 6.24–6.26).

After removal of the loose flange, any resin left on the tooth surface may be polished away (Figure 6.25d,e). If caries has taken hold, it should be removed and, provided it is not too extensive, the resultant cavity may be restored with a glass-ionomer cement or composite resin (Figure 6.26c).

The same procedure may be adopted with the so-called 'hybrid' resin-bonded bridge where one retainer is a conventional crown and the other a resin-bonded flange. Invariably, due to unequal retention between flanges, failure is more likely to occur in the attachment with the weaker retention, in this case the resin-bonded flange; this may be cut away and the rest of the bridge left as a cantilevered unit.

If the situation warrants the removal of the entire bridge, eg when an intermediate flange is involved, a number of commercial bridge removers may be used. These may employ either a falling weight or an actuated spring mechanism (Figure 6.27). A recent instrument uses a spring-loaded handpiece driven by a dental micromotor (Figure 6.28). The bridge must be supported with the free hand while the bridge remover is being used. A loop of dental floss may also be applied to secure the bridge (Figure 6.28b,c).

Great care must be taken when using these mechanical devices, particularly where auxiliary grooves and pins are present, because there is a danger that the enamel layer or even the whole tooth may be ruptured in the process. An instrument designed to lessen the damage caused to the tooth is the KJ Cavitron Insert (De Trey/Dentsply) supplied as straight and curved tips to be used in an ultrasonic scaling machine (Figure 6.29). The high-frequency vibrations are believed to disintegrate the resin–metal bond, thus allowing the flanges to be prised off easily (Jordan et al, 1986). There appears to be both cohesive failure within the resin and adhesive at the resin–metal interface with no apparent damage to the margins of the flange (Krell et al, 1988).

Macro-retained bridges, such as the perforated Rochette bridge or the mesh and bead types in the anterior arch, are the simplest to remove; often it is only necessary to give a sharp tap with a mallet on the handle of a straight chisel placed under the incisal margin in order to dislodge the flange.

Any resin remaining on the tooth surface may be ground down level with diamond stones. The abutment tooth may be re-etched as usual and the bridge bonded in place. New resin has a good affinity for old, refreshed resin and a secure bond should be established without difficulty.

Any caries present should be excavated and the defects restored as previously described. There should be no problems rebonding a bridge to either a glass-ionomer or a composite resin restoration if this is feasible.

If all else fails . . .

If the bridge persistently debonds, in spite of taking every care, then recourse to a conventional bridge or removable partial denture should be considered. It is a consolation that at least some, if not all, the abutment teeth (provided they are not ravaged by caries) would be reasonably sound to provide strong foundations for the new appliances.

Appendix I

Aspects of adhesion

In scientific parlance, adhesion is specific and limited by its definition and therefore cannot include union of materials through mechanical factors. In dentistry, this rigid definition poses considerable difficulties because good retention, clinically, is apparently achieved mainly through mechanical forces and with no assistance from molecular attraction. Furthermore, it is difficult to see, given the intrinsic microscopic roughness of all surfaces including teeth, how adhesion can be achieved solely by molecular attraction. Williams and Cunningham (1979) have proposed a more realistic definition: 'the state in which two surfaces are held together by interfacial forces, which may consist of forces of molecular attraction or mechanical forces.' When uncertain, the term 'bonding' may be preferred because it describes an 'observed situation' and does not involve specifying the mode of retention.

Adhesion theory is complex and abstruse; however, in order to appreciate both the demands made on a dental adhesive and the clinical steps necessary to implement successful bonding, some understanding of adhesion theory is essential.

Terminology

Confusion arises when terms are used without due regard to their precise meaning. Often terms such as 'adhesion' and 'bonding' or 'conditioning' and 'etching' are used in an arbitrary fashion. The following definitions may be found in the *British Standard Glossary of Dental Terms* (1983).

Adhesion

Adhesion is the physical force that attracts certain molecules at the surfaces of different materials when these are brought into contact. This is in contrast to *cohesion* which is the attraction between similar molecules within the same substance.

Adhesive

An adhesive is a material that joins other substances by adhesion.

Bonding

Bonding is a general term describing the joining of adhesives to a surface, or adherend. It does not define the mechanism of attachment.

Bonding agent

A bonding agent is a thin film of liquid painted over the surface of the adherend to enhance the adhesion of the applied material.

Bonds

Bonds are the forces of adhesion, which may be physical or chemical and vary in strength. Physical bonds are very powerful and are considered to be sufficient for most adhesive applications outside dentistry. Chemical bonds, however, are the most powerful forces of molecular attraction. They are usually more resistant than physical bonds to degradation by water—an important consideration in the moist conditions of the mouth.

Etchant

An etchant is an acid solution which at the appropriate concentration can partially decalcify tooth substance.

Etching

In dentistry, etching is the use of an acid solution to demineralize partially a selected area of tooth substance so altering its surface topography and providing micromechanical retention for certain types of restorative material.

Conditioner

A conditioner is a solution, usually of a weak inorganic acid, that will provide a clean surface for bonding. In clinical practice, 'conditioning' means gentle scrubbing of the enamel or dentine surface with the acid solution for a few seconds both to remove debris and 'grease' and to improve the attractive nature of the surface; consequently, when a fluid adhesive is applied it will spread completely over this surface—a process known as 'wetting'. This process does not imply any change in surface topography, and it falls just short of etching.

By definition, the role of an adhesive is to join two substances through adhesion. For this to occur the adhesive must be able to form an adhesive bond between the surfaces of the two substances which will hold them together. Thus, it acts as an intermediary performing in a way that neither adherend can, ie, by covering the surfaces thoroughly and effectively and then setting hard to form a mechanically sound layer (interface).

As noted above, adhesion in dentistry may involve two basic categories as shown in Diagram 1.

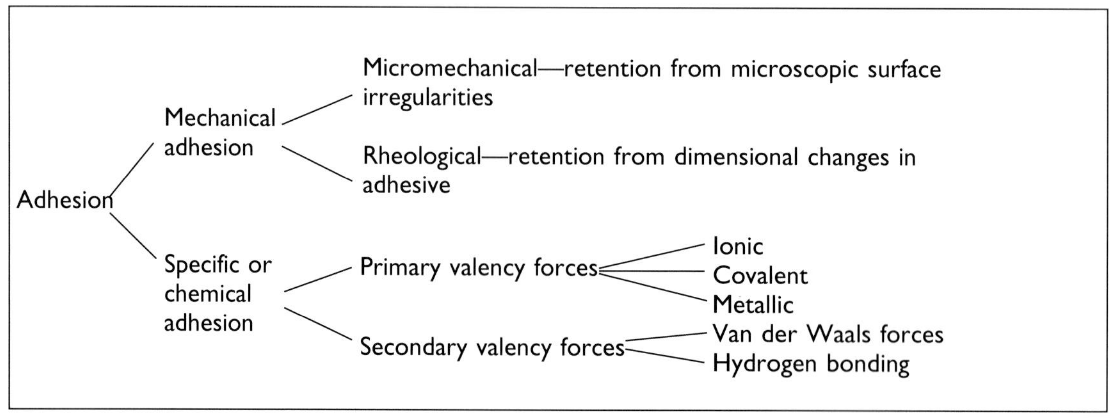

Diagram 1

Adhesion categories.

Mechanical adhesion

In surfaces that can be etched, such as tooth enamel and some metal alloys, minute irregularities may be produced. Provided the adhesive is able to penetrate these irregularities completely, very strong bonds may be formed. These bonds are especially resistant to shearing or 'sliding' stresses but their ultimate strength depends very much on the cohesive strength of the adhesive and of the substrate (adherend). In other words, to be of any practical value the interface bonds should be the last to fail in the event of mechanical disintegration of the substrate–adhesive system.

Dimensional changes due to expansion or shrinkage occurring during the setting of the adhesive, or due to rapid fluctuations in temperature, may assist or reduce mechanical retention. Unfortunately, most of the adhesive resins used in resin-bonded bridges tend to exhibit polymerization shrinkage when establishing stronger cohesive bonds. However, if the resin is applied as a thin film, less polymerization shrinkage may occur and any loss in mechanical retention will be insignificant.

By close adaptation of the adhesive to the substrate, intermolecular attraction (specific adhesion) can be developed or enhanced. These forces tend to be predominantly of the van der Waals type and are sufficient to form joints stronger than the cohesive strength of the adhesive and adherend. However, in certain circumstances, such as when conditions are severe during chewing or in extremes of temperature and a moist environment, chemical bonding (ie, hydrogen bonding) at the interface may be of more importance and may be required to augment van der Waals forces.

Primary valency bonds (see Diagram I) are extremely strong and may be seen in processes such as soldering and welding where metallic bonds form across the interface. In dentistry, such bonds are not normally prevalent although some adhesives may form primary bonds with the various components of enamel and dentine.

Criteria for effective adhesion

In addition to participating in one or more of the different modes of adhesion, the ideal adhesive should be able to:

1. Spread easily and completely over a surface, ie, it should show good 'wetting' properties.
2. Solidify (set) with minimal dimensional change so that excessive stresses do not build up during the union.

Surface phenomena and wetting

The extent to which an adhesive will wet a surface depends on the following factors:

1. The viscosity of the adhesive.
2. The surface topography of the substrate.
3. The surface energy of the substrate.
4. The presence of contaminants.

Viscosity

Viscosity is a measure of the ability of a fluid to resist relative motion within itself, ie, a measure of its consistency or ability to flow. Thick treacle has a high viscosity whereas a freely flowing liquid such as water has a low viscosity. Gross irregularities on very rough surfaces tend to impede the flow of liquids, and so on such surfaces the viscosity is of greater importance than on very smooth surfaces. Voids created by the inability of the fluid to permeate the surface often cause loss of adhesion.

Surface topography

Because adhesion to tooth surfaces is mainly by mechanical interlocking, it follows that the rougher the surface, the greater the surface area of contact. Here it must be emphasized that microscopic and not macroscopic roughness is the key factor. The latter which may be visible to the naked eye does not contribute to any significant increase in surface area of contact and, indeed, may create large pools of adhesive that are not always conducive to low setting shrinkage. Etching with a weak inorganic acid is the most effective way of increasing the microscopic roughness of the enamel surface.

Surface energy

Molecules within an ideal homogeneous solid or liquid are attracted equally to all their neighbours and are in a state of equilibrium. However, as they approach the surface there is a net inward pull back towards the larger numbers of molecules there, so creating a state of tension; there is also a tendency for different areas of the surface to separate—as though an elastic film had been stretched over the surface. This surface tension is evident in the formation of the meniscus of a liquid in a glass tube. With solids, it is rather more difficult to conceive of a surface tension in the same way and it is impossible to measure directly the free surface energy of a solid. However, by observation of the behaviour of a drop of liquid on the surface this energy may be demonstrated and indeed measured indirectly. The angle formed between the surface of a liquid drop and the adherend surface is called the *contact angle*, and it is measured at equilibrium. The contact angle is dependent on the surface tension of the liquid and the surface energy of the adherend and determines the degree of wetting that occurs. In general, low contact angles may be seen in low surface-tension liquids on high surface-energy solids and they result in complete wetting. Most domestic and industrial adhesives, eg epoxy resins, have low surface tensions. Conversely, it is difficult to bond anything to materials with an exceptionally low surface energy such as Teflon (polytetrafluoroethylene, PTFE) because very high contact angles result, with poor wetting and, therefore, poor adhesion. Such is the principle of the non-stick frying pan.

In dentistry, the situation is more complex. When microscopic roughness is required in enamel for enhancement of adhesion, it is important that the adhesive can permeate the capillary pores created by etching. For this to occur the adhesive must have a reasonably high surface tension—as we know from elementary physics, the height to which a liquid rises in a capillary tube is directly proportional to its surface tension. Williams and Cunningham (1979) have suggested that the best results should be achieved when the surface tension of the adhesive is high enough to encourage flow into the substrate irregularities, but not higher than the critical surface tension of that substrate.

Appendix II

A comparison between Panavia EX and Geristore

A study on the shear strength of resin-bonding agents used with cast metal restorations was recently reported by Reilly and co-workers (1991). Cast discs of nickel–chromium alloy were sandblasted with aluminium oxide grit and then applied to prepared enamel surfaces on extracted human molar teeth with each of the following resins: Comspan (LD Caulk), Panavia EX (Kuraray), Geristore (Den-Mat) and Gold Link (Den-Mat). All the specimens were stored for 24 hours at 37°C and then half the specimens were subjected to several cycles of thermal stress to simulate conditions in the mouth.

The average force in megapascals (MPa) required to shear off the specimens from the tooth surfaces was recorded as follows:

Comspan	1.29 MPa	Gold Link	1.54 MPa
Geristore	1.60 MPa	Panavia EX	2.94 MPa

Panavia EX appeared to provide greater shear strength for bonding to non-precious alloys such as Ni–Cr than to any of the other resins tested.

In-house testing by the Den-Mat Corporation gives a slightly different picture. The average values (in MPa) for shear tests after storage in water for 24 hours were as shown in Table 1.

Material	Gold	Non-precious metal	Stainless steel	Amalgam
Geristore	9.70	9.34	20.44	8.41
Infinity	11.23	11.82	18.73	6.50
C&B MetaBond	7.50	10.28	15.22	5.10
Panavia EX	3.11	9.34	10.91	3.65

Table 1

Infinity (Den-Mat) is the luting version of Geristore with a finer film thickness and a longer working time. Both Geristore and Infinity are dual-curing, ie, a snap-set polymerization reaction with light curing and a more gradual acid–base reaction of the glass-ionomer component, the latter reaction being termed 'infinite cure' by the manufacturers. C&B MetaBond (Parkell) contains 4-META resin, and Panavia EX is a phosphonated methacrylate resin. Besides being easier to use, Geristore/Infinity also scores over the other two resins because each has the ability to leach fluoride almost indefinitely.

Bibliography

Aboush YEY, Jenkins CBG (1987), Resin-bonded bridges: chairside methods of cleaning metal surfaces contaminated with saliva, *Br Dent J* **163**: 227–30.

Aker AA, Aker JR, Sorensen SE (1979), Effect of methods of tooth enamel preparation on the retentive strength of acid-etch composite resins, *J Am Dent Assoc* **99**: 185–9.

Ante IH (1926), The fundamental principles of abutments, *Mich State Dent Soc Bull* **8**: 14–23.

Atta MO, Smith BGN, Brown DA (1987a), A comparison of chairside and laboratory etching techniques for cast and bridge retainers, *Restorative Dent* **3**: 11–12.

Atta MO, Smith BGN, Brown DA (1987b), A comparison of electrolytic and non-electrolytic etching techniques for direct bonded bridge retainers, *Restorative Dent* **3**: 129–30.

Atta MO, Brown D, Smith BGN (1988), Bond strengths of contemporary bridge cements to a sand-blasted or electrolytically etched nickel–chromium alloy, *Dent Mater* **4**: 201–7.

Atta MO, Smith BGN, Brown D (1990) Bond strengths of three chemical adhesive cements adhered to a nickel–chromium alloy for direct bonded retainers, *J Prosthet Dent* **63**: 137–43.

Barkmeier WW, Shaffer SE, Gwinnett AJ (1986) Effects of 15 vs 60 second enamel acid conditioning on adhesion and morphology, *Oper Dent* **11**: 111–16.

Barrack G (1984), Recent advances in etched cast restorations, *J Prosthet Dent* **52**: 619–26.

Batchelder KF, Richter RS, Vaidyanathan TK (1987), Clinical factors affecting the strength of composite resin to enamel bonds, *J Am Dent Assoc* **114**: 203–5.

Bates D, Retief DH, Jamison HC (1982), Effects of acid etch parameters on enamel topography and composite resin–enamel bond strength, *Pediatr Dent* **4**: 106–10.

Bowen RL (1963), Properties of a silica reinforced polymer for dental restorations, *J Am Dent Assoc* **66**: 57–64.

Brady J (1986), Dry Tips: An improved aid to saliva control and measurements, *Dent Update* **13**: 329–34.

Brannstrom M, Nordenvall KJ (1977), The effect of acid etching on enamel, dentin, and the inner surface of the resin restoration: a scanning electron microscopic investigation, *J Dent Res* **56**: 917–23.

The British Standards Institute (1983), *British Standard Glossary of Dental Terms,* BS4492 (The British Standards Institution, London).

Buonocore MG (1955), A simple method of increasing the adhesion of acrylic filling materials to enamel surfaces, *J Dent Res* **34**: 849–53.

Burgess JO, McCartney JG (1989), Anterior retainer design for resin-bonded acid-etched fixed partial dentures, *J Prosthet Dent* **61**: 433–6.

Caputo AA, Gonidis D, Matyas J (1986), Analysis of stresses in resin bonded fixed partial dentures, *Quintessence Int* **17**: 89–93.

Chow LC, Brown WE (1973), Phosphoric acid conditioning of teeth for pit and fissure sealants, *J Dent Res* **52**: 1158.

Clyde JS, Boyd T (1988), The etched cast metal resin-bonded (Maryland) bridge: a clinical review, *J Dent* **16**: 22–6.

Creugers FF NHJ, van't Hof MA (1987), Treatment times for adhesive bridges, *J Oral Rehabil* **14**: 371–7.

Creugers NHJ, Snoek PA, Vogels ALM (1988), Overcontouring in resin-bonded prostheses: plaque accumulation and gingival health, *J Prosthet Dent* **59**: 17–21.

Creugers NHJ, Snoek PA, van't Hof MA et al (1990), Clinical performance of resin-bonded bridges: a 5-year prospective study. Part III: failure characteristics and survival after rebonding, *J Oral Rehabil* **17**: 179–86.

Deubert LW, Jenkins CBG (1982), *Tooth-coloured filling materials in clinical practice* (Wright PSG, Bristol) 109–13.

Eick JN, Johnson LN, Fromer JR et al (1972), Surface topography: its influence on wetting and adhesion in a dental adhesive system, *J Dent Res* **51**: 780–8.

Elderton RJ (1971), A modern approach to the use of the rubber dam, *Dent Practit* **21**: 3–23.

Eshleman JR, Moon PC, Barnes RF (1984), Clinical evaluation of cast metal resin-bonded anterior fixed partial dentures, *J Prosthet Dent* **51**: 761–4.

Fleming HB (1981), The FABB technique, *Dent Practice* **19**: 1–5.

Gottlieb EW, Retief DH, Jamison HC (1982), An optimal concentration of phosphoric acid as an etching agent. Part I: Tensile bond strength studies, *J Prosthet Dent* **48**: 48–51.

Gwinnett AJ (1981), Acid etching for composite resins, *Dent Clin North Am* **25**: 271–89.

Hamada T, Shigeto N, Yanagihara T (1985), A decade of progress for the adhesive fixed partial denture, *J Prosthet Dent* **54**: 24–9.

Hansson O (1989), The Silicoater technique for resin-bonded prostheses: clinical and laboratory procedures, *Quintessence Int* **20**: 85–99.

Haywood VR, Kanoy BE, Bruggers KJ et al (1990), Thermal removal of composite resin: effect on rebonding etched metal, *J Prosthet Dent* **63**: 289–91.

Hero H, Ruyter IE, Waarli ML et al (1987), Adhesion of resins to Ag–Pd alloys by means of the silicoating technique, *J Dent Res* **66**: 1380–5.

Hill GL, Zidan O, Gomez-Martin O (1986), Bond strengths of etched base metals: effects of errors in surface area estimation, *J Prosthet Dent* **56**: 41–56.

Hopkins C (1981), An immediate cantilever Rochette Bridge, *Br Dent J* **151**: 292–5.

Hudgins JL, Moon PC, Knap FJ (1985), Particle-roughened resin-bonded retainers, *J Prosthet Dent* **53**: 471–6.

Hussey DL, Pagni C, Linden GJ (1991), Performance of 400 adhesive bridges fitted in a restorative dentistry department, *J Dent* **19**: 221–5.

Ibsen RL, Strassler HE (1986), An innovative method for fixed anterior tooth replacement utilizing porcelain veneers, *Quintessence Int* **17**: 455–9.

Jedynakiewicz NM, Cunningham J, Williams DF (1985), Acid-etching and the fracture of rubber dam clamps, *Br Dent J* **159**: 121–3.

Jones ML, Richards BH (1984), The bonded bridge: an improved model? *Br Dent J* **157**: 138–40.

Jordan RD, Krell KV, Aquilino SA et al (1986), Removal of acid-etched fixed partial dentures with modified ultrasonic scaler tips, *J Am Dent Assoc* **112**: 505–7.

Karlsson S (1986), A clinical evaluation of fixed bridges, 10 years following insertion, *J Oral Rehabil* **13**: 423–32.

Kayser AF (1981), Shortened dental arches and oral function, *J Oral Rehabil* **8**: 457–62.

Kellett M (1987), The etch-retained metal restoration in hospital clinical use, *Br Dent J* **163**: 259–62.

Krell KV, Jordan RD, Denehy GE (1988), SEM analysis of ultrasonically debonded acid-etched metal retainers in teeth, *Am J Dent* **1**: 67–70.

LaBarre EE, Ward HE (1984), An alternative resin-bonded restoration, *J Prosthet Dent* **52**: 247–9.

Livaditis GJ (1986), A chemical etching system for creating micromechanical retention in resin-bonded retainers, *J Prosthet Dent* **56**: 181–8.

Lynch E, Tay WM (1989), The rubber dam in dental practice. In: Tay WM, ed. *General dental treatment* (Churchill Livingstone, London) Chapter 4.1.6/7.

Lynn AMJ (1987), Etch retained bridges, *Dent Pract* June 18.

Lyttle HA, Louka AN, Young J (1986), A study of the consistency of etch patterns on samples of various alloys as fabricated by commercial dental laboratories, *J Dent Res* **65**: 532, abstract 11.

McLaughlin G (1981), Composite bonding of etched metal anterior splints, *Compend Contin Educ Dent* **2**: 279–83.

McLaughlin G (1986), *Direct bonded retainers* (JB Lippincott Co., Philadelphia).

Moon PC (1987), Bond strengths of the lost salt procedure: a new retention method for resin-bonded fixed prostheses, *J Prosthet Dent* **57**: 435–9.

Musil R, Tiller H-J (1984), *The adhesion of dental resins to metal surfaces. The Kulzer Silicoater technique* (Kulzer & Co. GmbH, Wehrheim).

Myers DR, Butts MB (1985), Surface topography of the cavosurface enamel bevel following acid etching in primary teeth, *J Pedod* **10**: 63–7.

Nixon GS (1963), Dental problems of the brass-instrumentalist, *Br Dent J* **115**: 160–1.

Pameijer JHN (1985), *Periodontal and occlusal factors in crown and bridge procedures* (Dental Center for Postgraduate Courses, Amsterdam) 17–34.

Peutzfeldt A, Asmussen E (1988), Silicoatings: evaluation of a new method of bonding composite resin to metal, *Scand J Dent Res* **96**: 171–6.

Posner BT (1985), The uses of light activated composite resin in emergency situations in general practice, *Dent Practice* **23**(2): 1–3.

Reilly BE, Xy Yu, Davis EL et al (1991), Shear strength of resin bonding agents used with cast metal restorations, *J Dent Res* ***390***: abstr 993.

Reuter JE, Brose MO (1984), Failures in full crown retained dental bridges, *Br Dent J* **157**: 61–3.

Roberts DH (1970), The failure of retainers in bridge prostheses, *Br Dent J* **128**: 117–24.

Rochette AL (1972), Adhésion per polymères et traitement de surface en odontostomatologie, *Actual Odontostomatol* **98**: 175–231.

Rochette AL (1973), Attachment of a splint to enamel of lower anterior teeth, *J Prosthet Dent* **30**: 418–23.

Saunders WP (1984), The retentive impact strengths of various designs of resin-bonded bridges to etched bovine enamel, *Br Dent J* **156**: 325–8.

Shaw MJ, Tay WM (1982), Clinical performance of resin-bonded cast metal bridges (Rochette Bridges), *Br Dent J* **152**: 378–80.

Silverstone LM (1978), *Preventive dentistry* (Update Books, London) 97–132.

Silverstone LM, Hicks MJ, Featherstone MJ (1985), Oral fluid contamination of etched enamel surfaces: an SEM study, *J Am Dent Assoc* **110**: 329–32.

Simonsen RJ, Thompson VP, Barrack G (1983), *Etched cast restorations: clinical and laboratory techniques* (Quintessence, Chicago).

Simonsen RJ, Tierney CL (1985), SEM analysis of human enamel after variable acid treatment, *J Dent Res* **64**: 245, abstract 633.

Smith BGN (1990), *Planning and making crowns and bridges*, 2nd edn (Martin Dunitz, London).

Stokes AN, Tidmarsh BG (1986), Porous metal coatings for resin-bonded systems, *J Prosthet Dent* **56**: 170–5.

Stokes AN, Tidmarsh BG (1987), Porous metal coating—a microretentive alternative to etched metal prostheses, *Quintessence Int* **18**: 675–7.

Taleghani M, Leinfelder KF, Taleghani AM (1987), An alternative to cast etched retainers, *J Prosthet Dent* **58**: 424–8.

Tay WM, Shaw MJ (1979), The Rochette adhesive bridge, *Dent Update* **6**: 153–7.

Tay WM (1986), A classification and assessment of composite retained bridges, *Restor Dent* **2**: 15–22.

Tay WM (1987), Composite retained bridgework. In: Derrick DD, ed. *The dental annual 1987* (Wright, Bristol) 246–60.

Thayer KE, Doukoudakis A (1981), Acid-etch canine riser occlusal treatment, *J Prosthet Dent* **46**: 149–52.

Thompson VP, Del Castillo E, Livaditis GJ (1981), Resin bond to electrolytically etched non-precious alloys for resin-bonded prostheses, *J Dent Res* **60**: 377, abstract 265.

Veen JH van der, Krajenbrink T, Bronsdijk AE et al (1986), Resin bonding of tin electroplated precious metal fixed partial dentures: one-year clinical results, *Quintessence Int* **17**: 299–301.

Veen JH van der, Jongebloed WL, Dijk F et al (1988a), SEM study of six retention systems for resin-to-metal bonding, *Dent Mater* **4**: 266–71.

Veen JH van der, Bronsdijk AE, Slagter AP et al (1988b), Tensile bond strength of Comspan resin to six differently treated metal surfaces, *Dent Mater* **4**: 272–7.

Wada T (1986), Development of a new adhesive material and its properties. In: Gettleman L, Vrijhoef MMA, Uchiyama Y, eds. *Proceedings of the international symposium on adhesive prosthodontics* (Academy of Dental Materials, Chicago) 9–18.

Walker ML, Vann WF (1984), In vitro comparison of primary incisor enamel surfaces etched with an acid solution or acid gel, *Pediatr Dent* **6**: 203–13.

Williams DF, Cunningham J (1979), *Materials in clinical dentistry* (Oxford University Press, Oxford) 66–86.

Williams VD, Thayer KE, Denehy GE et al (1989), Cast metal, resin-bonded prostheses: a 10-year retrospective study, *J Prosthet Dent* **61**: 436–41.

Williams W, Drennon DG, Silverstone LM (1982), The effect of retainer design on the retention of filled resin in acid-etched fixed partial dentures, *J Prosthet Dent* **48**: 417–23.

Wiltshire WA (1986a), Tensile bond strengths of various alloy surface treatments for resin bonded bridges, *Quintessence Dent Technol* **10**: 227–31.

Wiltshire WA (1986b), Resin bonded fixed partial dentures utilizing additional pin retention, *Quintessence Int* **17**: 343–7.

Wiltshire WA, Ferreira MR (1987), A classification of resin-bonded bridges based on the evolutionary changes of the different technique types. *Quintessence Dent Technol* **11**: 253–8.

Yamashita A, Yamani T (1986), Adhesion bridge, background and clinical procedure. In: Gettleman L, Vrijhoef MMA, Uchiyama Y, eds. *Proceedings of the international symposium on adhesive prosthodontics* (Academy of Dental Materials, Chicago) 61–77.

Index

References in *italic* are to figures.